Sports, Body and Health vol. 7

The Essence of Sport

Verner Møller
&
John Nauright (eds.)

The Essence of Sport

University Press of Southern Denmark

© The contributors and the University Press of Southern Denmark 2003
Set and printed by Special-Trykkeriet Viborg
Cover design by UniSats
ISBN 87-7838-764-7

Cover photo: Danish football supporters (Polfoto).

University Press of Southern Denmark
Campusvej 55
DK-5230 Odense M

www.universitypress.dk

Costumers in the United States and Canada please contact:

International Specialized Book Services
5824 NE Hassalo St
Portland, OR 97213
Phone: 1-800-944-6190

www.isbs.com

Contents

Introduction   7

CHAPTER 1
Verner Møller:
What is Sport: Outline to a Redefinition 11

CHAPTER 2
John Nauright:
Nostalgia, Culture and Modern Sport 35

CHAPTER 3
Henning Eichberg:
Three Dimensions of Playing the Game: About Mouth Pull,
Tug-of-War and Sportization 51

CHAPTER 4
John Bale:
A Geographical Theory of Sport 81

CHAPTER 5
Niels Kayser Nielsen:
Scandalous Sport: Finland as a Case Study 93

CHAPTER 6
John Hoberman:
"A Pharmacy on Wheels": Doping and Community Cohesion
Among Professional Cyclists Following the Tour de France
Scandal of 1998 107

CHAPTER 7
Allen Guttmann:
Ideal Types and Historical Variation 129

Introduction

This anthology developed out of a seminar held at the University of Southern Denmark – Odense, on the 15th of November 2000, hosted by the Institute of Sports Science and Clinical Biomechanics and organised by Verner Møller, associate professor of sports studies at the Institute.

At this time John Nauright, a sports studies scholar, was at the University of Southern Denmark as a visiting professor in the Institute of Sports Science and Biomechanics. As luck would have it, the International Federation of Sports Journalists was concurrently holding a conference in Copenhagen called "Play the Game, Reaching for Democracy in Sports," dealing with the corruption of modern sport in its various aspects. Professor John Hoberman was in attendance as an invited speaker. Hoberman's widely recognised research in sports studies had been of great importance to Møller, who had just finished a research project on the doping scandal that almost destroyed the 1998 Tour de France. Most of this work was carried out while he was on sabbatical at Keele University, where the sports geographer John Bale holds a chair.

The Tour scandal raised questions about the future of elite sport in a particularly urgent way. In the media one heard claims that rampant drug use might well mean the end of modern sport. These claims were, however, quite puzzling, in part because "sport" itself was never defined by those predicting its demise.

At Keele, Bale and Møller had often discussed the current state of elite sport, and this led to reflections about the nature of sport itself. While Møller suggested that developments in modern high-performance sport were best understood in term of aesthetics, Bale maintained that the neutral and standardised nature of sport spaces meant that sport was better understood as a scientific enterprise. It goes without saying that this discussion was not, and has never, been finally resolved.

Stimulated by the many offences committed by athletes against the ethical ideals of sport, our discussions made it clear that old-fashioned questions about the essence of sport were not nearly as obsolete as they were often held to be. Typical explanations of the problems that afflict modern sport are (1) that they are caused by a few cynical cheaters who exploit sport for their own benefit; (2) that they are due to the fact that modern athletes in general demonstrate morally corrupt attitudes that damage sport as a subculture; and (3) that they are a consequence of the growing economic stakes in the sports business that stimulate greed and induce managers and sponsors to hype the superhuman feats of their athletes. If we do not feel that these familiar explanations really address the current predicament in which sport finds itself, then it would appear that the question of the essence of sport requires some thoughtful reexamination.

With Hoberman and Nauright in Denmark, Møller could not resist the temptation to try to arrange a seminar on this topic. Bale accepted an invitation and proposed that Niels Kayser Nielsen also be called upon, because he knew that Nielsen's wry approach to sports always ignites debate. The idea was to see what would happen when scholars from different countries addressed themselves to a question that seems to be important to all those who share a scholarly approach to sports. From an academic standpoint, this involved a certain risk in that straightforward answers to such questions would certainly not be forthcoming. When Henning Eichberg, another participant in "Play the Game," heard that a seminar on the essence of sport would take place in Odense a day later, he too promised to show up. Throughout his long career, Eichberg has produced an extensive body of work that takes a cultural relativist approach to sports. Hence it was obvious that he too should be on the panel.

Each panel member gave a fifteen-minute presentation, after which the floor was open. The participants engaged in lively debates. Afterwards, people who had attended the seminar asked if the papers were available. Most presenters, however, had spoken from notes, which had made possible a spontaneity that greatly enlivened the discussion. For this reason, there were no papers to hand out. There was general agreement, however, that the speakers would write formal papers that would then be sent to Professor Allen Guttmann for his comments. We are especially grateful to Professor Guttmann for taking upon himself the twin roles of arbiter and commentator.

We would also like to thank John Hoberman, who besides writing his own article has done a tremendous job enhancing the linguistic quality of papers by the non-native English-speaking contributors. Furhermore we would like to acknowledge Jørgen Povlsen, the head of the Institute, for the support he gave to the seminar. Without his financial assistance neither the seminar nor this book would have been possible. Finally John Nauright would also like to thank Jørn Hansen for arranging the invitation to come to Denmark, thereby enabling him to contribute to this seminar and to the production of this volume.

We hope these papers will reinvigorate the debate about the nature of modern sport. Indeed, the range of perspectives presented here ought to make this volume well suited to teaching sports studies to university students.

While some of these authors focus on broad topics and employ a variety of humanistic approaches, others make use of the case-study format to make their arguments. In the first chapter, Verner Møller begins the debate, as he did in the seminar, by setting the stage for an analysis of the essence of sport. Nauright then examines the ways in which sport is used to create cultural meaning, including how sports are remembered and reshaped in nostalgic recollection and in nostalgia-driven politics. Here he focuses on the English-speaking societies on which his own research has been based. Eichberg, in his usual eclectic fashion, then turns to mouth-pulling and other tugging games to discuss the sportifying of originally non-sportive types of physical culture. Bale, the internationally recognised doyen of sports geography, then outlines a spatial theory of sport in his ongoing battle with Møller about the roles of technology and uniformity in modern sport. Niels Kayser Nielsen provides us with unique insights into how sport is read through the lenses of sports scandals and national identity. Hoberman concludes this series of papers with a discussion of the doping crisis in professional cycling. Finally, Allen Guttmann, a pioneer in academic sports studies, puts these papers into a wider context that will encourage further debate. We conclude by noting that a great deal remains to be said and written about such a complex an issue as the essence of sport.

November, 2002   Verner Møller, Odense
                                                      John Nauright, Dundee

What is Sport:
Outline to a Redefinition

Verner Møller

Today, sport is an enormous global success story. Yet it is also supposed to be in a state of crisis. By the beginning of the twenty-first century, it has become clear that sport, which during the previous century became a global mass culture, is fundamentally different from what it has traditionally been thought to be. The ideological investments that have been made in sport by sports educators, officials, organisations and politicians have lost much of their authority. In the light of escalating drug abuse, accelerating commercialism and the constant effort to enhance the entertainment value of sports, it has become clear that the idea that sport is primarily a healthy and educational activity suitable for building character is impossible to maintain. There is no longer any doubt that the success of sport is based on its ties to market forces. This connection accounts for the fact that the traditional idea of sport is now in a critical condition.

Neo-Marxist sports criticism cannot explain this crisis. Nor can conservative sports idealism. It is therefore time to propose an alternative approach to the conceptualising of sport. Inasmuch as cultural relativism now seems like common sense to the great majority of scholars in the humanities, the idea of searching for an essence of sport may seem foolhardy. Indeed, the sheer variety of sport would seem to make this a hopeless task. On the other hand, those who pursue sports studies must assume that what we call sport can be understood through analysis. That is, the analyst must be confident that it is possible to interpret these activities. I would guess that even scholars who regard themselves as relativists can presume – after having carried out an analysis of, say, rugby – that they have said something essential about that particular sport. And if it is possible to scrutinise one sport, then it should be possible to analyse sports in general. This requires, however, a change of emphasis, from specific to common characteristics. In this context we cannot ignore what we have learned from Allen Guttmann's influential work: *From Ritual to Record. The Nature of Modern Sports* (1978), namely, that today's sport is not the same as in primitive or ancient times, but is rather a phenomenon that changes over time due to societal and cultural changes. For example, ascription was much more important than achievement in ancient contests that served as ritual practises closely linked to religion. We should, therefore, recognise that giving up the relativist approach will require a correspondingly rigid definition of sport. In other words, one must focus on sport as an ideal type in a Weberian sense. It is true, of course, that Weber was not an essentialist. On the contrary, he was, as a neo-Kantian, a nominalist who thought of the ideal type as a thought-construction that serves to grasp the reality from which the scientist is excluded. It can be argued, however, that the effort to map out the ideal type, in this case *sport*, does imply a will to capture some sort of essence. The basic assumption is that, although the meaning and figuration of sport is changing, there are still core elements that can be identified and applied advantageously to the search for an explanation of the current crisis in modern sport. It may be, as Guttmann claims, that modern sport can be characterised by secularism, equality, specialisation of roles, rationalisation, bureaucratic organisation, quantification, and the quest for records, but it is unlikely that these features are what attract athletes to participate and spectators to watch. Understanding the fascination and the allure of sport requires a change of focus from the spectacle – sport as event – to the inner motivations which make sport an expression of the human spirit.

Some semantic difficulties arise from the fact that the English term *sport* covers a wide range of phenomena, while the Scandinavian languages employ different words. In Scandinavian countries the term *sport* connotes what in English is referred to as competitive sports or high-performance sport, while sport-for-all is defined by the words *idræt* and *motion*. The latter refer to activities such as walking, jogging or riding a bicycle to work, all of which differ from the Scandinavian concept of *sport*. Henning Eichberg's trialectic model suggests that sport is not one thing but contains at least three different types of physical culture: (1) high-performance sport, which is driven by results and records; (2) exercise sport, which is motivated by the pursuit of fitness and recreation; and (3) sport for bodily experience and expression, where it is not the result but the process that is the motivation; examples would be creative dancing or tai chi chuan where the purpose is the experience of spirituality or sensuality. Eichberg thus identifies three kinds of sport: sport for production, sport for reproduction or recreation, and sport for creation. Although the model is an elegant thought-construction it is not intended to encompass all of the qualities of sport. Eichberg's macro-perspective model is thus too simple to account for the complex problems of today's sport. Let us reserve the term sport for the first category of the model.[1] Sport is far more complex than the model allows. There is no more reason to assert that sport is productive than to claim it is non-productive, or recreational, or creative, as I will argue throughout this chapter.

After this clarification it should be clear that a crucial feature of sport is the code of winning and losing. If winning is not the aim of the game, we are not talking about sport but about play or exercise. One can run, cycle, even play soccer for the sake of health. In that case sport is turned into a means to promote health and we are no longer talking about sport in the sense we have defined above. Sport is inextricably linked to a striving to win. It is worth noting that victory is not a product but a symbolic value expressed by medals, laurels, points and status. The latter points to the fact that sport is hierarchical in its structure. Sport means the pursuit of excellence and striving to be the best. Consequently, sport is by nature elitist.

This chapter responds to the paradoxes of sport by proposing an approach which deals with them as different expressions of a certain logic that is inherent in the sportive context. That is to say, this chapter is based on the idea that it is, in fact, possible to identify the core elements of sport and thereby grasp its essence. If that does not take us directly to the essence of sport, it should at least serve to deepen our understanding of what sport is all about. Before I argue how sport can be understood as an aesthetic phenomenon, I will point out some exemplary fallacies and mis-interpretations in neo-Marxist sports criticism, and then make some critical remarks about the idea that sport is primarily an educational project, as is claimed by the sport idealists.

Sports criticism

Humanistic sports research only began to develop in the 1960s. It originated primarily as a critique of sport based on neo-Marxism. This emancipatory doctrine analysed modern sport employing a critique of industrial capitalism and its mechanisms of exploitation (Morgan 1994). By analogy with labour in capitalist societies, sport was seen as subjugated to the tyranny of abstract time and space and was understood as a sinister but effective tool to teach people to accept, and even appreciate, the rigid time and space disciplines of industrial society. In a similar fashion, setting records was seen as a celebration of capitalist profit-seeking, and thereby a tribute to an alienating ideology of growth.

Pointing to the immense effort invested in training by legendary stars like the runner Emil Zatopek and the swimmer Mark Spitz, one of the most influential of the Marxist sports critics, Jean-Marie Brohm, gives the following explanation of why the 'Ecole Emancipée' is against high-performance sport: "Sports training is thus structurally similar to production line work in a factory and involves the same inhuman work pace" (Brohm 1978:68). This analogy is typical of the early sport criticism. Although it is thought-provoking, it is nevertheless imprecise. It is based on the fallacy that, because sport shares certain characteristics with work, it *is* essentially work. This is no more than an argument by analogy.

Having said that, it must be stressed that Marxist sport criticism was accurate in pointing out the special character and logic of sport. For example, Brohm settles accounts with the common assumption that sport is a valuable pedagogical tool to promote virtues like fair play and sportsmanship. Looking at the lines along which modern sport has developed, he writes:

> The reality of sport is not as rosy as is often made out. In every field people are beginning to realise the price paid for success in the medals race. Everywhere people are wondering about the human, educational, cultural and political consequences of the hunt for new records, of the frantic drive for biological output and of nerve-racking physical challenges. The unease caused by this painful questioning of sport's perspectives contributes to the crisis. "Just how far can top-level competitive sport go?" Will not the many deviations suffered by sport sooner or later lead to its complete degeneration? (Brohm 1978:14).

Today, a quarter of a century later, the same argument is often presented in different media, and the reasons for this are clear. Sports salaries and prize money are spinning out of control. Drug problems are escalating. Tournaments and the number of games played are constantly being expanded. The demands on elite athletes are steadily growing. The physical and psychological pressures on athletes produce many problems. Disabling injuries, alcoholism and other kinds of abuse, even death, are prices that an increasing number of athletes have to pay for their careers. It appears that sport has fallen into a moral abyss.

The woman behind the doping revelations at the Tour de France 1998, the Minister of Youth and Sports and Communist Marie-Georges Buffet, justified her heavy-handed intervention in the doping scandal by saying that such measures were necessary for the purpose of carrying out real reform. As a responsible politician she did not have any alternative, since this action was necessary to protect the riders, she claimed. In an interview with the Danish newspaper *Politiken* she expressed her view of the riders. She said that she regarded the stars as workers who were in the clutches of money-grubbing sponsors and sports directors. "Most of the riders are very well paid, but their careers are short, they usually stay uneducated all their lives and their health is at risk", she said. At two points during the tumultuous 1998 Tour the riders demonstrated their disapproval of these measures by going on strike. Buffet claimed that she fully understood their actions, but she was surprised by the reasons given by the riders. Their tactics were not aimed at their employers, those who in her opinion had initiated and managed the drug abuse: sports directors, physicians and sponsors. On the contrary, they were aimed at the police and the press, who in their different ways supported the minister's initiative. Her comment on this sounded almost like an echo of Brohm: "The problem is the riders' false consciousness" (*Politiken*, 7 September 1998). In other words, she suggested that the riders were mentally incompetent and unable to understand what would serve them best in the long run.

The minister's arrogant exclusion of the possibility that drug use could be a free choice of autonomous men is not the only interesting point here. It is also worth paying attention to the construction of the story, about athletes as powerless prey who are deluded by superior agents, a story which is essential if such interventions into the lives of athletes are going to be accepted by public opinion. If it were not for this story there would be no basis for the intervention, which can otherwise be thought of as a matter of judgment. The minister has presumably sensed that her construction is essentially baseless. Otherwise she would not have commented as she did on the fact that the riders earn princely salaries. By pointing out that their careers are short and that most of them will stay uneducated for the rest of their lives, she confirms her view about the heartless exploitation of the riders. Their short period of stardom is dearly bought. Over the longer term the athletes are actually being impoverished.

Considering the professionals' earnings – a top rider's annual salary is far beyond an ordinary skilled worker's aggregate lifetime earnings – the idea of impoverished riders is hard to maintain. This problem involved in such analogical thinking is already evident in Brohm's critique of elite sports. Using skiing as an example, he shows how sport degenerates on account of the constant striving to achieve new records. Industry invests in research to improve the quality of the equipment. Streamlined suits and high-tech skis make skiers go faster and faster, and the risk increases accordingly. Brohm refers to the production of a 'phantom-suit' so smooth that a skier who fell slid at high speed and was in great danger until he eventually hit something. It took a serious accident to get this suit banned, and Brohm argues that even this did not really put an end to this dangerous development:

> The maximum and average speeds reached in the down-hill events are steadily increasing: 75, 80, 90 m.p.h. At Cervina, in Italy, maximum speeds of up to 125 m.p.h. have been clocked up. So it should come as no surprise that the list of top-level skiers, seriously injured or killed on the 'field of battle' for a few dollars (or rather medals) more grow steadily longer. This absurd, inhuman obsession with winning is not limited to skiing (Brohm 1978: 17).

Brohm's description invites a comparison with ordinary working men Coal miners, for example, put their lives in danger to earn 'a few dollars'.

The difference is that skiers (and even boxers) are not driven to compete by the same economic necessity that drives the miners. Many of them participate because they are attracted to the competition. The contest is the motivation, and that is incomprehensible from Brohm's perspective. He does not make the slightest attempt to understand the special attractions that lure athletes to sports. He simply avoids the question by calling it an absurd obsession. He just continues to cite examples, including the corruption of rugby. To be sure, he has a point when he says:

> However, those who sing the praises of this noble sport can no longer conceal the fact that the risks of the game are on the increase and accidents are becoming alarmingly frequent – an awkward fact for a 'game' which is supposed to be 'educative' (Brohm 1978: 17).

Although Brohm denounces athletes' motivations for competing, he is on the mark when he points out the weakness of the sports idealists' position. The idea that sport is ennobling is, it would seem, false. On the contrary, it seems reasonable to argue in favour of the opposite: Sport contains the seeds of violence and moral decay. The idea that sport is fundamentally a good thing derives from the fact that, rooted in the traditional folk games, it was adapted and civilised by the leisure class and thereby connected to the ideal of the gentleman.

Sport as a matter of education

Sportsmanlike conduct is not, however, a natural form of behaviour. Sportsmanlike conduct is not a consequence of sport but of a discipline that is strong enough to prevent acting out certain impulses that can be stimulated by competitions (Grupe: 1975). Precisely because sport does not call for moderation, but, as Baron de Coubertin already realised, encourages *excess*, it is useful for educational purposes in that it promotes self-moderation and self-control. The scepticism that sport encountered on the European continent can be seen as a presentiment, or even an early understanding, of its destructive potential. In Germany and Scandinavia a disciplinary physical culture like gymnastics preceded the arrival of sport. Swedish gymnastics in particular was organised according to scientific principles, in line with the ideas of its originator, Pehr Henrik Ling (see Ling 1866).

Adherents of the Swedish system in Denmark argued that German gymnastics was merely acrobatic, promoting an impressive animal agility at the expense of a rational, harmonious, and healthy development of the body. Adherents of German gymnastics claimed that the Swedish system was too limited and that gymnasts were better off with the challenge of the inspiring German model. For this reason their attitude to sport was quite positive, while 'the Swedes' felt that it presented a dangerous threat to the harmony of body and soul.

From the educational perspective of Ling's gymnasts, sport was completely irrational. To be sure, it was restricted by certain rules, but there were no rules prescribing a rational logic to its movements. Its lack of purposeful grace and ideal carriage seemed irresponsible and even chaotic. The Danish Director of Gymnastics, K.A. Knudsen, offered his own critique in *On Sport – Impressions of a Journey in England* (1895). While in England he attended, among other events, a high jump competition between Englishmen and Finns, where he noticed a striking difference in style. While the Finns ran straight towards the bar and finally jumped right up, landing properly on their legs, the Englishmen slanted towards the bar, doubled up in the jump, and eventually landed on both hands and feet. According to Knudsen, they expended too much energy in their jumps. Although the Englishmen jumped the highest, their style was, in his view, unworthy of emulation. What he witnessed led him to draw the following conclusions:

> The English do not regard gymnastics as a tool to educate the body as a whole but as sport, and by sport the English mean the idea of competition. The point Ling made; that one exercises for one's own purposes and not to be compared with others, is remote from the English way of thinking. All their work devoted to bodily development is turned into competitions about who can be the best. The aim of their gymnastics is not the development of beauty, health and the highest degree of working ability, but a number of tricks performed with the most impressive perfection (Knudsen 1895: 20).

For Knudsen, who was totally absorbed in the continental tradition of a restrictive body culture, it was difficult to see any pedagogical value in sports. The problem from his point of view was that the focus on winning excluded any other purpose. Sport does not, like gymnastics, function primarily to serve other purposes. It is, so to speak, a prodigious waste of time, energy and resources.

Sport, as Knudsen experienced it, was practised by men of culture, to be sure, but that did not convince him that it was an effective way to create gentlemen. As sport spread the amateur ideal came under increasing pressure, and the discrepancy between claims about sport's character-building qualities and how sport was actually practised grew wider. This was also recognised in the birthplace of sport. Even the noble sport of cricket was subjected to a scandal at the Ashes-tournament in 1932 (Williams 1999). The Englishmen had gone to Australia to win. The host country, however, presented a very strong team which included the legendary batsman Donald Bradman. The captain of the English team,

Douglas Jardine, had decided to employ controversial tactics to gua-
rantee success, which outraged the record crowd of 50,962 cricket fans.
Jardine had instructed his 'big guns', Harold Larwood and Bill Voce, to
practice 'bodyline' bowling, aiming at the body instead of at the wicket.
This strategy created havoc among the Australians, as the ball came
screaming at the batters at speeds of up to 145 km/h.

Some of the Australian players who did not hit the ball got hit themselves. The crowd became enraged, and especially so when the Australian
captain fell to the ground after being hit on the temple. In these circumstances Jardine elected to return to the traditional mode of play after an
over or two.

Nevertheless, the damage was done, in that the ideal of sport had been
clearly violated. Jardine's bodyline tactics were regarded as a threat to
the very spirit of sport. The press mourned the death of truly magnani-
mous competition. Even the political situation was influenced by the
episode, as trade relations between the two countries were called into
question.

In that day and age it hurt to see sport show its true face. Today, however, this face has become all too familiar. Of course it is aggravating to
see Diego Maradona breaking the rules by using his hand to outwit Peter
Shilton. But this kind of situation no longer causes genuine outrage. At
most, it makes fans impatient with the 'blindness' of the referees. The
world has become used to winning as the rationale of sports. Hence only
the naïve, or those who can take political or economical advantage of
moral posturing, will nowadays advocate sport on the basis of its moral
qualities.

Sport and morality: The Tour de France scandal

This may seem like a bold assertion regarding the public's response to the
Tour de France scandal. All of the media, after all, expressed their disapproval. Yet it is worth noting that the loudest voices in the choir were
mainly politicians and certain other parties with vested interests in the
event: sports officials, journalists, and sponsors. Nor are their motives
hard to find. For the politicians, the scandal was an outstanding opportunity to present an ethical and responsible profile by promising they would
take all necessary steps to get rid of this odious practice and hunt down
the cheats and their associates. For those with direct economic interests
in cycling, the only thing to do was to limit the damage by playing to a
public opinion that has heard a great deal about sport's character-
building qualities. Yet suddenly it was evident that this propaganda was
little more than empty rhetoric.

Many sports officials, along with journalists with close connections to
the cycling world, praised Buffet's initiative, claimed they had long been

suspicious that something was amiss in the sport but that they had lacked evidence, and therefore kept silent. But what is going on when sports officials can suspect that doping is going on without taking steps to investigate it if they really think that drug abuse is unacceptable? And how can it be that journalists can resist the temptation to investigate when they have a feeling there is a story under the surface?

The former professional-rider Paul Kimmage's book *Rough Ride* (1990), the winner of The William Hill Sports Book of the Year award, puts the lie to the sports journalists' assertion that there is an impenetrable *'omerta'*, a law of silence, which makes it impossible to persuade sources with inside information to speak out. The obvious explanation is that there is consent between riders, leaders and the press, which broke down under pressure from the authorities. It seems reasonable to assume that there is a silent acceptance amongst the interested parties that the show must go on and a common understanding that it could not continue – at least not at the same level – without the use of stimulants. The sanctimonious attitude that most of the European press presented in its crude smear campaign against cycling, without any attempt to understand the doping issue, was probably a result of a fear of public opinion and the threat to a lucrative sports business. The apparent irresolution of the sponsors suggests that this was the case. Festina, the sponsor of the team that caused the scandal in the first place, maintained their sponsorship. Other sponsors not directly involved in the affair, such as Rabobank, announced they would end their sponsorships immediately if they became aware of any drug abuse being practised by their teams.[2]

When those with vested interests in high-performance sports are clearly fearful and groping in the confrontation with the doping issue it is not because they are genuinely morally stricken by the fact that doping means cheating. It is not unsportsmanlike behaviour in a traditional sense that bothers them, but rather that it exposes their riders to medical risk. As a threat to health, doping is a violation of one of the foremost taboos of our time, and that is the reason why it is a much more serious offence than the cheating of which Maradona's famous goal has become an emblem.

The doping hysteria that descended upon the 1998 Tour de France can be compared with the public reaction to the bodyline cricket scandal of 1932. Indeed, we should not exclude the possibility that a pragmatic attitude towards doping will develop along with a tolerance for other kinds of cheating in sports. The current tendency towards a growing acceptance of drug taking among ordinary people makes this even more likely. In a world of plastic surgery, Prozac, Viagra, Rogaine and similar medical solutions to human desires, doping will easily be reinterpreted as a way to sustain or enhance human health, meaning that doping will no longer violate the modern ideals of health (Møldrup 1999). Hereafter the rationality of sport will be given free rein, and that will put an end to the illusion that sport is naturally compatible with morality and modesty.

The attraction of sport

If we must give up the idea of sport as inherently good; if, in other words, we can no longer legitimise sport by claiming its moral value, how then do we evaluate this phenomenon? What is the attraction of sport for athletes and spectators?

As shown previously, it does not seem epistemologically fruitful to elaborate on the sport-work analogy as an alternative to the idealistic point of view. This analogy disregards the fact that sport is basically a free choice. Nobody is educated to be a professional athlete, and only a small number of athletes get the chance to make a living from their sports. There are, however, a lot of amateurs dreaming about the opportunity to leave their jobs and take advantage of a professional career. If this were nothing more than athletes wishing for overnight wealth and economical security ever after, one might wonder why so many athletes continue their careers long after they have made their fortunes. There must be another explanation, and the reason why this has been difficult to find is that sport has been miscategorised. Leading sports critics have characterised sport in terms of standardisation and performance enhancement (e.g. Umminger 1962, Bale 2002). It is within this framework that the analogy with labour on the production line was invented (Hoberman 1984). By way of contrast, idealists have asserted that sport rightly belongs within the field of ethics. From this perspective, sport has benefited from being constructed as a positive social and political force; yet it is precisely this idealistic viewpoint that leads to sport's becoming an instrument of politics as soon as it violates the health taboo.

So what are the intrinsic attractions of sport? The apparent paradox is that the cultural importance of sport continues to grow even as it is accused of succumbing to moral decay. In his famous book *Homo Ludens: A Study of the Play-Element in Culture* (1938), the cultural historian Johan Huizinga writes:

> Play lies outside the antithesis of wisdom and folly, and equally outside those of truth and falsehood, good and evil. Although it is a non-material activity it has no moral function. The valuations of vice and virtue do not apply here.
>
> If therefore, play cannot be directly referred to the categories of truth or goodness, can it be included perhaps in the realm of the aesthetic? Here our judgement wavers. For although the attribute of beauty does not attach to play as such, play nevertheless tends to assume marked elements of beauty. Mirth and grace adhere at the

outset to the more primitive forms of play. In play the beauty of the human body in motion reaches its zenith. In its more developed forms it is saturated with rhythm and harmony, the noblest gifts of aesthetic perception known to man. Many and close are the links that connect play with beauty (Huizinga 1949:6).

It is indisputable that sport is one of the most developed forms of play in modern culture. Therefore, following Huizinga, it seems obvious to suggest that sport must rightly be understood as a phenomenon belonging to the realm of aesthetics. This change of perspective helps to explain why athletes' are willing to take risks for insignificant amounts of money. We also come closer to comprehending the enhanced cultural significance of sport despite its moral decline.

Although one can practise sport for a living, as in the case of the arts, it is qualitatively different from work and education in that it does not serve any external purpose. It is, like art, an expression of human surplus and useless in an ordinary sense. It seems, in fact, that the sport-art analogy is more useful than the sport-work analogy. The attraction of sport has nothing to do with the rational calculations of everyday life. On the contrary, sport is tempting because it puts everyday life in brackets and creates its own world of meaning. Sport is not entirely remote from everyday life, but its premises are radically different. In sport the surplus expenditure of energy and risk-taking are seen as superior to accumulation and vigilance. In everyday life, the situation is the opposite. By presenting a charismatic alternative to everyday life, it becomes a potentially subversive practice. It is both an alternative order and a demonstration of the real power and special beauty of disorder. The rebels, magicians, and artists who in stunning moments alter conventional patterns and thereby change situations to their advantage can inspire us.

Given the peculiar futility of sport, the affection it inspires is rather strange, and it can appear that it serves the same needs and longings as religion. What we are talking about is, after all, an abstract world, even a non-world, a construction that at least to the uninitiated may seem completely senseless, but in which the initiated can find an alternative and meaningful dream world. In that respect it offers a kind of compensation for the loss of religious meaning in a secular age.

The sports sections of newspapers contain pages of results that are completely irrelevant to broad sectors of society. Yet they constitute important news for very large numbers of people. Sports fans spend long hours studying these pages carefully, calculating whether teams might win championships, etc. Although this news is generally irrelevant from a social perspective, to the initiated it provides a significance that can even be interpreted as a threat to society. This is already clear in that the sporting event, and the passionate engagement of the fans, appears to be a squandering of time and resources. Football hooliganism, for example, is a reminder of the connection between sport and the Dionysian side of human beings as well as a clear expression of the precariousness of this relationship.

In Marshall McLuhan's influential work, *Understanding Media: The Extension of Man* (1964), the idea is applied to the social function of play. McLuhan reminds us that play, which in tribal societies is appreciated as a way of expressing both collective and individual impulses, functions differently in an individualistic society. "Carried into an individualistic society, the same gambling games and sweepstakes seem to threaten the whole order of society" (McLuhan 1964: 235). He regards games as collective *reactions* to mainstream cultures and invokes the example of the ancient Olympic Games:

> Games are dramatic models of our psychological lives providing release of particular tensions. They are collective and popular art forms with strict conventions. Ancient and non-literate societies naturally regarded games as live dramatic models of the universe or of the outer cosmic drama. The Olympic Games were direct enactments of the *agon*, or struggle of the Sun god (McLuhan 1964: 237).

Accordingly, McLuhan understands art as an advance upon the dramatisation of games. Art became a sort of civilised pendant to magic games and rituals. Both forms were influenced by an increasing emphasis upon the individual, as people turned away from cosmic themes in favour of the psychological. McLuhan's dramatic argument, which for good reasons has inspired much criticism, is that: "The key to understanding the mind of primitive man is available in our new electric technology that is so swiftly and profoundly re-creating the conditions and attitudes of primitive tribal man in ourselves." (McLuhan 1964: 237) In modernity, too, play is to be interpreted as a way to stage the dramas of life and to add a necessary depth to existence. "The wide appeal of the games of recent times – the popular sports of baseball and football and ice hockey – seen as outer models of inner psychological life, become understandable." (McLuhan 1964: 237). Here McLuhan opens the door to an understanding of sport's revolutionary potential, in contrast to the neo-Marxist's idea of sport as an "opiate of the people". Yet he too seems puzzled by the reality of professionalism, and this prevents him from developing all of the implications of his argument:

> Art and games enable us to stand aside from the material pressures of routine and convention, observing and questioning. Games as popular art forms offer to all an immediate means of participation in the full life of the society, such as no single role or job can offer any

man. Hence the contradiction in "professional" sports. When the games door opening into the free life leads into a merely specialist job, everybody senses an incongruity (McLuhan 1964: 237).

McLuhan sees as clearly as Huizinga that sports belong to the field of aesthetics, and it is here that he finds their appeal and value. He also agrees that professionalism leads to the corruption of sport. This is all the more interesting in that their arguments on behalf of this thesis are diametrically opposed to each other. The conservative Huizinga argues:

> Now, with the increasing systematisation and regimentation of sport, something of the pure play-quality is inevitable lost. We see this very clearly in the official distinction between amateurs and professionals (or "gentleman and players" as used pointedly to be said). [...] In modern social life sport occupies a place alongside and apart from the cultural process. The great competitions in archaic cultures had always formed part of the sacred festivals and were indispensable as health and happiness-bringing activities. This ritual tie has now been completely severed; sport has become profane, "unholy" in every way and has no organic connection whatever with the structure of society, least of all when prescribed by the government. The ability of modern social techniques to stage mass demonstrations with the maximum of outward show in the field of athletics does not alter the fact that neither the Olympiads nor trumpeted international contests have, in the smallest degree, raised sport to the level of a culture creating activity. However important it may be for the players or spectators, it remains sterile. The old play-factor has undergone almost complete atrophy (Huizinga 1949: 199).

While McLuhan sees the separation between society and play in ancient cultures as an advantage, which melts away when sport is made professional and thus dragged into the whirlpool of capitalism, Huizinga, on the other hand, sees an essential organic relationship between society and play in former times that is severed by professionalism, and this development makes sport almost revolutionary.

Although both thinkers make valuable contributions to our understanding of sport, they are limited by a critical perspective which makes them see change as degeneration. It does not, in fact, seem logical that the role of money in sports should change the phenomenon fundamentally and destroy its valued characteristics. Various art forms were being supported by patrons long before professionalism in sports arose, and it is unlikely that anyone would claim that such arrangements altered and influenced those art forms in a negative way. And though it is true that some famous artists of the past lived impoverished and miserable lives, many artists today are making fortunes from their art. This is due to economic and societal developments, and who would posit a causal connection between poverty and great art? The crucial shortcoming of the critical perspective is that it sees change as decline. If we are to succeed in our attempt to understand current developments in sport in an unprejudiced way, we have to develop the insights of Huizinga and McLuhan. In what follows we will pursue the essence of sport by exploring the hypothesis that sport is first and foremost an aesthetic phenomenon.

Sports as aesthetics

In his book *The Body Language* Andrew Blake claims that

> there is no developed sense of sporting aesthetics; no sense of exactly what it is in sporting activity that gives either the participant, or the observer, so much pleasure; and no sense of the continuous importance of writing about sport as a part of "literature" (Blake 1996: 17).

In his famous essay on the Tour de France in *Mythologies* (1957), Roland Barthes carries out an analysis – reading the event as an epic – where he argues that the popularity of the Tour is due to the fact that it satisfies a human need for mythological meaning. That is, it offers a narrative for identification and interpretation of certain basic aspects of human life. One may wonder why Barthes' approach has not attracted more scholars working in the field of sports studies. According to Blake, one explanation for the lack of interest in reading sport as literature is the neo-Marxist hostility towards sport in general. He finds another and equally important explanation in C.L.R. James' classic *Beyond a Boundary* (1963), where

> James argues that the principal reason for the absence of sport from aesthetic theory is that both aesthetics and those who discuss aesthetic theories are elitist and that sports, especially as the elite see them, are popular. The elitism prevents people on both sides of the high/mass culture divide from seeing that sports belong in the same domain as theatre, ballet, opera and dance (Blake 1996: 194).

Nowadays popular culture has become a legitimate research field that is taken seriously by many scholars. Accordingly, interest in sports studies is growing. It is still a common assumption among the cultural elite, at least in Europe, that sport is a mass culture phenomenon that should not be paid much attention. Those who do are often called sports idiots. Similarly, those who work in sport studies are generally not the most respected in the academic world. They are usually academics educated in other disciplines who can be divided into two types. Some are former athletes who have taken up sport studies concurrently with more conventional research topics because they have a soft spot for sports and are interested in the development of the field. As a rule, they demonstrate a lot of insight, like an anthropologist who has lived a long time among the people who are the subjects of his or her study. Their views, however, are often influenced by nostalgia. Others have not been able, or fortunate enough, to launch university careers within their major areas but have found a niche in sport studies which enables them to nurse their academic ambitions. Their lack of interest in sports and low self-esteem that derives from working in a less prestigious area should not be underestimated as explanations of their lack of sensitivity to the quality of sport. It is hardly a coincidence that it is highly regarded scholars in prestigious disciplines, such as Huizinga, James, McLuhan, and Pierre Bourdieu, who invoke sport's relationship to aesthetics. Bourdieu called sport a kind of *l'art pour l'art* of the body in his opening lecture at the History of Sport and Physical Education Association (HISPA) meeting in 1978. And although he is clearly sceptical about the development of modern sport, throughout his lecture he does elaborate on this point, drawing parallels between sports and the arts. It is worth noting that he implicitly criticises the amateur ideal that Huizinga presents as the ideal attitude, as noted above. Bourdieu claims, to the contrary, that the doctrine of the amateur is one variant of an aristocratic philosophy that turns sport, like art, into a selfless activity (Bourdieu 1980).

How is it that these distinguished outsiders find it so obviously appropriate to inscribe sports in the field of aesthetics? One reason may be that they are fundamentally disinterested in sports. When outsiders define sport, it is usually because they find the phenomenon useful for casting light on another subject, such as the essence of cultural development as in Huizinga's case, or the societal consequences of the mass media that is the focus of McLuhan's analysis. Therefore, instead of focusing on the complexity and heterogeneity of sport, they are concentrating on certain of its features. That is, they are "instinctively" searching for the essence of sport, which, I believe, they would not have done if the analysis of sport had been their primary objective. A look at the basic features of sport will reveal why sport is so easily inscribed in the field of aesthetics and why it should be compared with art.

As mentioned above, sport exists in a dimension that is distinct from everyday life. It is dramatic and spectacular and thus appeals to a wide audience. According to Blake, certain sporting events are watched on television by a third of the world's population. Moreover, sport demands the pursuit of excellence. It is not like a craft you either can or cannot do. It is rather an endeavour that requires a constant striving towards perfection.

And without special gifts one cannot master a sport any more than one can master the violin without possessing a special talent.

The drive towards victory requires not only an immense amount of training but also a measure of inventiveness. What Knudsen took offence at when he witnessed the high jump competition in England was that the Englishmen used a new technique that was unfamiliar and did not suit the ideals of the "Swedish system". Therefore he regarded it as cheating, although it was a style corresponding to the logic of sport in so far as there were no rules against it and it was more efficient than the style practised by the Finns. The experience was obviously thought-provoking and had the potential to broaden Knudsen's perspective, yet another example of how comparisons to other phenomena in the field of aesthetics constantly appear. The style that Knudsen found inappropriate was not so different from the one Leni Riefenstahl portrayed in her famous documentary *Olympia*. Today the technique used at the 1936 Berlin Olympics appears somewhat awkward. We have now become used to the elegant 'flop style' introduced at the 1968 Mexico City Games by the American Dick Fosbury. Since the days when the Englishman Thomas Anderson's 1.60 meters was recorded as the world best, the run-up-and-jump style has been perfected by numerous changes, and the world record has been elevated to an impressive 2.45m by the Cuban Javier Sotomayor. The competitions we witness today still feature high and fascinating jumps. They are at the same time expressions of human efficiency, corporeal beauty and elegance of movement. It is remarkable that one consequence of the implicit striving toward victory in sport can enhance its aesthetic qualities. Other examples can be found in boxing, skiing and football. Icons like Muhammad Ali, Ingemar Stenmark and Pele all set new standards and improved the aesthetic quality of their sports. Their performances suggest that there is an invisible bond between beauty and efficiency. Strikingly, it is not just those sports where the aesthetic qualities play a central role, as is the case in figure skating, gymnastics, dance, platform diving etc., that are expressive and rhythmical and therefore intuitively recognisable as aesthetic.

Sport and purpose

The philosopher David Best endorses the idea that there is a coherence that unites aesthetics and efficiency. In his essay "The Aesthetic in Sport" he points to the grace of champion gymnasts like Olga Korbut and Ludmilla Tourisheva. Although their performances are extremely demanding, they demonstrate "such remarkable economy and efficiency of effort that it sometimes looks effortless" (Best 1979: 349). He actually compares the gymnasts' efficiency and precision with the textual economy of a poem, where superfluous words would in a similar manner detract from its aesthetic quality. But he does not accept the idea that sport is an aesthetic phenomenon. His argument is that the aesthetic quality of sports is merely incidental. According to Best, sport is basically purposive, and this even applies to an "aesthetic" sport like gymnastics. In his attempt to separate what he just has joined together so convincingly, he states:

> The poet may take liberties with the sonnet form without necessarily detracting from the quality of the sonnet, but if the gymnast deviates from the requirements of, say, a vault, however gracefully, then that inevitably detracts from the standard of the performance (Best 1979: 349).

This argument breaks down, however, in the case of Olga Korbut, who actually did exceed the known standards and got a vault named after her. In fact, many great gymnasts have invented new expressive elements and thereby transgressed the conventional forms, and the Fosbury flop reminds us that this can happen outside of gymnastics, as well. (This is one more problem for Best's argument.) Even when Best argues that sport is not an art form, he does so unconvincingly. He justifies his point of view as follows:

> it seems to me that even in those sports in which the aesthetic is intrinsic, and which are therefore intentionally performed to give aesthetic satisfaction, we cannot justifiably call them art forms. For in skating, diving, trampolining and gymnastics the performer does not have the possibility of expressing through his particular medium his view of life situations. It is difficult to imagine a gymnast who included in his sequence movements which expressed his view of war, or of love, or of any other issue. Certainly if he did so it would, unlike art, *detract* to the extent from his performance (Best 1979: 353).

While this is difficult to imagine, the fact is that it happens. The famous ice dancing couple Isabelle and Paul Duchesnay performed an impressive programme in 1991 that was explicitly inspired by a South American revolution, and it made a great impact. The expression of pain and emotional suffering certainly did not detract from their performance; in fact, they won the world championship. By coincidence I later watched a ballet based on exactly the same theme, similar costumes and an almost identical choreography. I assume that this ballet was the model for the ice dancers' performance, but in theory it might have been the other way around. Although the Duchesnays' performance is more recent than Best's article, the example seems to undermine his categorical distinction between art and sport. And one could add that even the idea of *l'art pour l'art* makes it problematic, in so far as we recall Bourdieu's idea that sport is the *l'art pour l'art* of the body. The doctrine of *l'art pour l'art* reminds us that art does not have to express a view of life or a political ideology. The easily identifiable problems of Best's argument derive from his central point, which is:

> the *manner* of achievement of the primary purpose is of little or no significance as long as it comes within the rules. For example, from the competitive point of view it is far more important for a football or hockey team *that* a goal is scored than how it is scored. In very many sports of this kind the overriding consideration is the achievement of an external end, since that is the mark of success (Best 1979: 346).

This view has been challenged in a striking essay by the philosopher Joseph Kupfer, in which he virtually reconceptualises sport. Kupfer criticises Best for basing his theory on popular opinion, when instead he ought to have begun his analysis by identifying the assumptions upon which the public's attitude is based. According to Kupfer, there is no point in using what "would-be professionals or partisan spectators" think for the purpose of understanding the nature of sport. What the majority believes should not serve as "the standard by which we judge what is in the nature of things or what is good" (Kupfer 1979: 357). Kupfer's search for the nature of sport takes him to the concept of play as the most appropriate point of departure. That is appropriate, in that the notion of play implies enjoyment. If you do not enjoy playing, you will stop. It is impossible to force anybody to engage in play which, following Huizinga, is characterised by its aimlessness. Kupfer's starting point is also plausible in that we also speak of sports as "playing a game", which involves participation for no other reason than the enjoyment of a challenge. Although one can practise a sport for monetary gain, it is false to claim that it is a primary feature of sporting activity. Originally, games have no purpose other than the delight taken in playing them. Introducing external purposes into sports is foreign to the games themselves.

In other words, although sport, like art, may be used as a means to an external end, this does not tell us anything essential about sport. By changing the perspective from extrinsic to intrinsic qualities, Kupfer is actually freeing the conception of sport from ideological and societal influences, thereby bringing the core of sport to the fore. Treating sport as a primarily aesthetic phenomenon thus makes possible a more coherent understanding of the entire phenomenon. Kupfer's argument is that the intrinsic striving for perfection is far more important for an understanding of the attraction of sport than results and record-breaking. In his view, results are signs of excellence rather than the defining criterion of sport. His argument deserves to be quoted at some length along with his explanation of the aesthetic qualities of sport:

> Playing well, then, is not external to the game, rather, it is the full realization of the activity. Scoring and winning are at once conclusions of play and the "natural" completion of excellent play; they are signs or evidence of such excellence. [...] In an attempt to show that competitive sports are "purposive" (serve an external end) a quasi-empirical appeal to what professional athletes and their audiences would or do value is made. This appeal is persuasive only because we have become inured to the fact that such valuation is itself based on ends extrinsic to sport. The force of reference to the importance of scoring to professional athletes or their audiences stems from the contingent connection between winning in sports and the attainment of "goals" external to the game itself such as financial or social gain. It is ironic that the *contingent* bearing of such extrinsic ends upon sport underlies the attempts to show that in competitive sport the play is *logically* subservient to its "extrinsic end" of scoring (or winning). We should not, then, take current practice or attitude toward competitive sports as the criterion for locating scoring in the logic of sport (Kupfer 1979: 358).

Having refuted the commonly held view of sport as purposive, Kupfer continues by emphasising the intrinsic features that suggest that the overriding value of sports, and not least competitive sports, is aesthetic. So he claims that "economy and efficiency of effort are accomplished in movement, which is continuous and fluid: sport provides us distinct balletic values." (Kupfer 1979: 358). These characteristics are especially accentuated in non-competitive "form sports," even though aesthetic qualities emerge from other sources such as tension, co-ordination, cohesiveness and balance that come to the fore in competitive team sports. Drama is a key element of competition. The excellence of the athlete is defined in relation to his team as well as his opponent. In the game, contending wills clash with each other to form a whole. Each participant does everything to gain the upper hand, thereby forcing the opposition to do the same, so that the total performance can reach a kind of perfection. As Kupfer expresses it:

> As in art proper, the antagonism between part and whole is overcome. The part is brought to full development through its reciprocal relations with the other parts (members). Concepts such as timing, jelling, flowing, harmonizing, and executing attest to this aesthetic ideal in competitive sport. [...]
> *Temporally extended opposition* is the significant aesthetic addition

competition provides. The aesthetic objects such opposition offers range in scope and duration. We delight in a movement, play, rally or drive, a sub-unit of the game such as inning, (golf) hole, or quarter, as well as a game, series of games, or an entire season. The game itself no doubt is the most typical as well as accessible object of appreciation. Movements and plays, rallies and drives combine to create crucial foci of tension amidst stretches of relative respite. The game is the wider dramatic context for momentary movement: the body moves to the rhythm and tempo of the whole.

Repetitions, balance, pace, variations, crescendoes and decres-cendoes conspire to flavor a game with a rhythm and correlative mood or atmosphere. Some games are tense, stingy encounters in which defense dominates and scores are hard earned as if squeezed from a resistant world. Others are sprawling, brawly affairs, scoring barrages threatening to last forever. [...] It is appropriate, moreover, to speak of games in the "expressive" or "emotive" idiom typical in description of art works: games may be "grim," "breezy," "jovial," "solemn," "lively" and so on. As with works of art, games can fail to fill out into discernible wholes possessed of strong aesthetic quali-ties. Some games never seem to find a rhythm and in others dramatic tension is all but dissipated in early scoring or lackadaisical play; the latter mars the beauty of a game by destroying the rhythmic element dependent upon the crispness of execution (Kupfer 1979: 358).

One may object that Kupfer – although his exposition is cogent in its premises – falls into a trap of assumed agreement on terms. (Lowe 1977). It is indisputable, however, that he, having changed the perspective from extrinsic to intrinsic qualities, clears away obstacles to an understanding of what at first appears to be an incomprehensible sporting practice. It therefore seems worthwhile to use his article to rethink sport from within and attempt to explain its challenge to decorum. It may be useful to regard sport as an *oeuvre* and, consequently, as an essentially aesthetic phenomenon. If we accept that the athlete's attraction to sport is of the same kind as the artist's attraction to art, and thus become reconciled to the idea that the motivation for engaging in sport is the opportunity it provides for self-expression, we find that some of the apparent paradoxes of sport vanish. The conundrum Brohm left unresolved, namely, that skiers would risk their lives for money or medals, can now be resolved, as will the mysterious fact that amateurs too are willing to risk their health on behalf of hazardous jumps, breakneck descents or potentially dan-gerous drug-taking. When sport is regarded as a drama in which athletes perform on the basis of an inner drive or passion, there is no need for a materialist explanation of their behaviour. There is no reason to continue the pointless condemnation of athletes' behaviours, since this change of perspective makes it clear that drug-taking and dieting that results in anorexia are simply regrettable side-effects rather than the result of corrupted characters. These are side-effects comparable to those found amongst musicians and ballet dancers, poets and other artists, who do whatever is necessary to create their sublime works and then find themselves trapped in serious abuse or self-destructive behaviours.

The essence of sport – a conclusion

My motivation for suggesting that sport should be understood as a fundamentally aesthetic activity is neither to defend sport in its time of crisis nor to play down the serious nature of the side-effects mentioned above. Explanations that posit economic motives are clearly inadequate, and a moralizing attitude can only serve to encourage self-righteous' indignation and condemnation. My other purpose is to try to understand the voluntary risk-taking of elite athletes. When we focus on the aesthetic qualities of sport we realise that passion is another of its crucial features, which is why spectators are so passionate about sport, because passion is contagious.

As soon as we have accepted that sport contains an element of passion, we are in a position to understand sport from within. And from this point of view it is tempting to claim that it is actually possible to say something about the essence of sport. If we hesitate, it is because we realise that an essence is not concrete. It is only manifested in how athletes think about what they do. Accordingly, we cannot define sport on the basis of the characteristics of the activity, so that, for example, football and swimming are sports whilst the Inuit game of mouth pulling is not. In fact, what makes swimming a sport is that swimmers ascribe meaning to the competition beyond the time they are actually competing. Ascribing meaning to championships, and the ambition that makes one want to become a champion, are typical characteristics of the sporting spirit. Thus some sort of organisation and institutionalisation is a prerequisite for calling competitions sport. So if two people decide to race from one street light to the next for the fun of it, they may reveal a competitive spirit that is not, however, identical to the sporting spirit. This does not exclude the possibility that mouth pulling and other tug-and-pull games might be classified as sport.[3] The Japanese Sumo may serve to show that an activity does not have to be indigenous to the West or internationally recognised to count as a sport. That certain activities develop into sports with global appeal, while others do not, may be due to differences in aesthetic potential and in their respective abilities to satisfy needs for identification, mythological meaning, and their potential for symbolizing important aspects of life. In secular times these common human needs can no longer be satisfied by religion. So sport, which in ancient times was bound up with religious ritual, can now become an *ersatz* religion, creating a narrative of its own that features heroes and villains, Gods and Devils – a narrative whose manifest appeal is rooted in its transcendence of the mundane limitations of everyday life.

Notes

1. It is worth noting that Eichberg's former colleague Ejgil Jespersen, who was actually the first to suggest this tripartite model, labelled the second category "Idræt" as welfare" and the third category as non-sport. Ejgil Jespersen: "Redaktionelt," in *Centring* 1981/3-4 p. 97-98). For this reason, I think it is legitimate to exclude these alternative movement cultures from the concept of sport. Their inclusion will only serve to blur genres, while the topic here is sport in its typical form, which, it must be emphasised, does not mean understanding sport in terms of a stereotype.
2. What in the first place looks like indecisiveness on the part of the sponsors seems on closer inspection to be a consequence of different but carefully prepared marketing strategies. When Marc Streel – a star of the most successful and ambitious Danish team: Home/Jack & Jones (today CSC-Tiscali) – was caught in 1999 when a blood test revealed a haematocrite value above 50 percent – an indication that he had been using the banned drug EPO – he was immediately dropped from the team. The team remained, however, a serious contender for cycling's first division, which means access to the big races like the Tour de France, which in turn gives the sponsors value for their money. Nevertheless, the real-estate agency Home gave up their part of the sponsorship as a consequence of this episode, while the clothing company Jack & Jones decided to continue. There seem to have been rational calculations behind both decisions. Home chose a high moral profile in spite of the team's good prospects, stating that they are in a business where high ethical standards are essential. The survival of Jack & Jones, on the other hand, depends on their ability to connect a certain lifestyle to their products, and the exposure through cycling may be effective – perhaps even more with doping than without it. Hence they backed the team until the contract expired, even though a second embarrassing doping case occurred. The Danish social-democratic newspaper *Aktuelt* decided to stop their coverage of professional cycling until the doping problem was solved. In doing so, the paper supposedly demonstrated its categorical rejection of doping. The move seemed somewhat peculiar, however, in that the newspaper continued cover to cover other sports as usual, thereby encouraging the illusion that sports other than cycling present clean competitions. The paper's strict moralistic attitude is, in my opinion, a dubious one.
3. See Henning Eichberg: "Three Dimensions of Playing the Game. About Mouth Pull and Other Tug" in this anthology.

References

Bale, John (2003). "A Geographical Theory of Sport" in Verner Møller and John Nauright eds.: *The Essence of Sport*, University Press of Southern Denmark.

Barthes, Roland (1970 (1957)). *Mythologies*, Paris, Seuil.

Best, David (1979). "The Aesthetic in Sport" in Ellen W. Gerber and William J. Morgan eds.: *Sport and the Body: A Philosophical Symposium*, Philadelphia, Lea & Febiger.

Blake, Andrew (1996). *The Body Language – the meaning of modern sport*, London, Lawrence & Wishart.

Bourdieu, Pierre (1980). *Questions de sociologie*, Paris, Les Edition de Minuit.

Brohm, Jean-Marie (1978). *Sport – A Prison of Measured Time*, London, Ink Links.

Eichberg, Henning (2002). "Three Dimensions of Playing the Game. About Mouth Pull and Other Tug in Verner Møller and John Nauright eds.: *The Essence of Sport*, University Press of Southern Denmark.

Grupe, Ommo (1975). *Grundlagen der Sportpädagogik*, Schorndorf.

Guttmann, Allen (1978). *From Ritual to Record. The Nature of Modern Sport*, New York, Columbia University Press.

Hoberman John M. (1984). *Sport and Political Ideology*, Austin, Texas, University of Texas Press.

Huizinga, Johan (1949 (1938)). *Homo Ludens: A study of the Play Element in Culture*, London, Routledge & Kegan.

Jespersen, Ejgil (1981) "Redaktionelt" in *Centring* 1981/3-4.

Kimmage, Paul (1990). *Rough Ride – Behind the Wheel with a Pro Cyclist*, London, Yellow Jersey Press.

Knudsen, K.A. (1985). *Om Sport – Indtryk af en Rejse i England*, Copenhagen.

Kupfer, Joseph (1979). "Purpose and Beauty in Sport" in Ellen W. Gerber and William J. Morgan eds.: *Sport and the Body: A Philosophical Symposium*, Philadelphia, Lea & Febiger, 1979.

Ling, P.H. (1866). *Samlade Arbeter*, vol. 3., Stockholm.

Lowe, Benjamin (1977). *The Beauty of Sport: A Cross-Disciplinary Inquiry*, New Jersey, Prentice-Hall, Inc., Englewood Cliffs.

McLuhan, Marshall (1964). *Understanding Media: The Extension of Man*, New York, McGraw-Hill.

Morgan, William J. (1994). *Leftist Theories of Sport: A Critique and Reconstruction*, Urbana and Chicago, University of Illinois Press.

Møldrup, Claus (1999) Den medicinerede normalitet, Copenhagen, Gyldendal.

Umminger, Walter (1962). *Helden, Götter, Übermenschen*, Düsseldorf, Econ Verlag.

Williams, Jack (1999). *Cricket and England: a Cultural and Social History of the Interwar Years*, London, Frank Cass.

Nostalgia, Culture and Modern Sport

John Nauright

If you build it, he will come...
The thrill of the grass...
Ease his pain...
People will come...
Baseball is part of what was once good in America and could be again...
Dialogue from "Field of Dreams"

Sport is one of the most significant shapers of collective or group identity in the contemporary world and is a powerful force in virtually every society. Often sporting events and people's reaction to them are the clearest public manifestations of culture and collective identities in a given society. Frequently, sport is inscribed with the power to liberate and elevate the human spirit – to create moments of escape from the mundane. For many people sports and major sporting events form important parts of their collective and individual identity and they are integral to their ways of seeing the world around them.

In this chapter I explore sport as a cultural and nostalgic activity. Though sport has become increasingly just another form of commodified culture serving the interests of global capitalism and media empires, at its essence lies a power based on the joy and expression of human skill and athleticism. Great achievements, victories and performances provide the raw materials of individual and collective memories and connections between the past and the present. Paul Connerton (1988: 3-17) suggests that consciousness, identity and collective memory are generated through commemorative ceremonies and in bodily practices. Through such practices, images of the past emerge that legitimate a present social order. Events, like Cup Final Day or Super Bowl Sunday, generate collective cultural experiences linked to sport. A. Barlett Giamatti (1989) passionately argued that sport goes further in producing moments:

> when we are all free of all constraint of all kinds, when pure energy and pure order create an instant of complete coherence. In that

instant, pulled to our feet, we are pulled out of ourselves. We feel what we saw, become what we perceived).

It is a moment when something not modern but ancient, primitive – primordial – takes over. It is a sensation not merely of winning, for the lesson of life is that you cannot win, no matter how hard you work, but of fully playing: as the gods must play, as whoever is not us – call it the Diety or History or whatever is Untrammeled – must play, complete, coherent, freely fulfilling the anticipated fullness of freedom (1989: 35).

Michael Novak (1974: xii), writing some years before Giamatti agrees with this approach. He argues that the "basic reality of all human life is play, games, sport, these are the realities from which the basic metaphors for all that is important in the rest of life are drawn". Giamatti further argues that it is the memory of such moments that bring us back again and again in the attempt of recreating or recapturing such moments of freedom and release. While many take a less idealistic view of sport it is clear that it is a potent cultural force in modern society.

What I mean by "sport" needs to be made clear before moving forward. Sport is the form of body movement culture that is focused on achieve-ment in a competitive environment, as opposed to other forms of bodily movement such as dance, play, games or recreation. Modern achieve-ment sport requires winners and losers as well as great performers. It is also primarily a spectatorial and cultural experience that became global in scope during the twentieth century. Sport also is a highly nostalgic practice as the remembering and reconstruction of past achievements and glories of an individual or team are powerful cultural activities.

Sport provides key sites for the production of nostalgic led nationalism promoted by politicians and business leaders to serve their wider political and economic interests. Additionally, sport operates nostalgically at local levels and many communities of fans seek to maintain local identity through their sporting teams and the collective memories of past per-formances (see for example, Phillips & Nauright, 1999; Robson, 2000). I address the nostalgic impulses modern sport generates and the political use of sporting nostalgia in examining the broad role of sport in modern society using case studies from the United States and New Zealand and discussion of nostalgia in the face of global corporatisation of sport. Nos-talgia lies at the heart of sport's cultural role in society and memories of sport, – though with the pain often remaining – as much as the perform-ances themselves, are the real essence of sport.

Sport, Nostalgia and Culture

There have been many ways of reading and inscribing sport in a cultural sense. Many people in the United States would argue that baseball is the essence of America or American culture as demonstrated in the ethnographic research of Charles Springwood (1995). Fathers bring their sons (and sometimes mothers and daughters are involved) from all over America, and indeed other countries, to "play catch" on the field where the film *Field of Dreams* was shot. In the process they feel that they are making new connections across generations and with their own sense of Americanness. While this is certainly not universal, it is representative of a belief in the redemptive power of a particular sport that transcends its mere formal competitive on field practice. In the English context, Anthony Bateman (2002) argues that the literature of cricket that emerged during the nineteenth century literally "wrote" the game into existence as an idealised sporting and cultural form that came to be representative of the essence of Englishness. This literature was marked almost from the outset with nostalgic longings of youth and pastoralism developing during and after the 1830s as England entered a period of rapid industralisation and urbanisation. More recently, Nick Hornby's *Fever Pitch* similarly literaturises association football and cultural attachments formed around it as the game sought to reposition itself during the 1990s after the hooligan troubles of the 1970s and 1980s.

In examining sport in society, one useful theoretical starting point has been to analyse sport in the context of hegemony and hegemonic struggle as Richard Gruneau, John Hargreaves and others did during the 1980s and early 1990s (Gruneau, 1983; 1993; Hargreaves, 1986; Ingham & Loy, 1993). Hegemony is an ongoing process of accommodation and apparent compromise – the winning of "consent". Despite its usefulness in helping us understand the ways that power is negotiated and how certain cultural forms emerge, hegemony often keeps us focused at the structural level and does not go far enough in explaining how a person as a person experiences life and changes to identity. One way around this apparent impasse is to combine structural analysis with that of the individual life course in attempting to unravel why people respond to changes or threats in particular ways. Nevertheless, we cannot totally disentangle individuals from the societies and cultures in which they exist. Individual memory is always formed in relation to social or collective memory, meaning that the production and selection of memories are developed through processes of interaction between the individual and society.

In seeking to move beyond more structural analyses of the relationship between past and present in the shaping of identities, nostalgia is useful as an explanatory tool. Nostalgia, or the longing for a happier and simpler past, provides people with a coping mechanism to face the rapidly changing world. The ways in which we remember the past are integral to our experiences of the present. While the past itself may indeed be "a foreign country" as historian David Lowenthal (1985) asserts, our conceptions of it pervade our everyday lives. We engage with the past to give us a sense of security in the present or to guide us in shaping our future. Increasingly, the past has been used in a nostalgic sense to provide us with a sense of who "we" are as individuals and as members of society. Nostalgia confronts us every day from our longings for the "good old days" to our sense of insecurity in a world changing faster than many of us can comprehend. In such times of rapid social, cultural and political shifts, people frequently draw on elements of their past cultural identity in order to cope with societal changes. They often retreat into nostalgic recollections and reconstructions of a happier past time when their world was more stable and organised (see Davis, 1979) and when they had more individual or collective power. As DaSilva and Faught (1982:49) argue, "Nostalgia requires a collective emotional reaction toward, if not an identification with, a symbolisation of the past".

Nostalgia also helps link group with individual identity as remembering past events operates at both individual and societal level. As Kathleen Stewart following the work of Susan Stewart states, nostalgia "in positing a 'once was' in relation to a 'now' it creates a frame for meaning, a means of dramatising aspects of an increasingly fluid and unnamed social life" (Stewart, 1988: 227). Taking the concept further, Lowenthal (1985) argues that nostalgia "can also shore up self-esteem, reminding us that however sad our present lot we were once happy and worthwhile ... nostalgia is memory with the pain removed. The pain is today". Nostalgia can also be used by dominant power groups to legitimate their position thorough promoting a sense of cultural security through cultural practices common to many members of society. People also utilise nostalgia to challenge new ways of thinking promoted by political and cultural elites.

The nostalgic use of sport and the history of sport has been one of the most significant areas in the process of sustaining identities and solidarity through shared experiences of heroic deeds in specific societies. In most societies, major sports events have been imbued with significant cultural power and relevance as evidenced by politicians' haste to be seen with sporting heroes or at major sporting events. Many years ago, Robert Lipsyte in *Sportsworld: An American Dreamland* (1975) demonstrated how sport had enveloped wider American society in the Nixon era and had become central to public culture and political practice. In Ronald Reagan's America, the nostalgic representation of sport was a prominent element in the President's efforts to create a warm and secure feelings about American society and history. In Britain former Prime Minister John Major adopted this approach with his referrals to the Village Green and cricket as quintessentially English. In Australia, Prime Minister John Howard led moves to link sport, war, the Sydney Olympics, the centenary of Australian Federation and support for the monarchy in mobilising a nostalgised vision of the Australian past and of Australian culture.

In order to better understand the role of sport as a cultural phenomenon and a powerful political tool, we need to examine closely just how
sports and sporting events present and past are used to sustain, or in
some cases, create identities for particular political purposes. As my own
research experience has concentrated on English-speaking societies, the
examples I discuss are limited in scope to the USA, Australia, Canada,
England, New Zealand and South Africa. As Matti Goksøyr has shown,
though, the nostalgic impulse in sport transcends language and cultural
barriers at least within Europe (Gøksoyr, 1998). Nostalgic uses of sport
have served a conservative purpose in political initiatives to shore up
hegemonic social values and preserve remnants of past glories in the face
of immigration, changing values, and in South Africa, a new political
system. At times, present inadequacies in sports or other spheres are constructed with reference to the once more "glorious" past thus creating a
feeling that if a society is not great now, at least it once was great and perhaps could be again if older ideals were somehow reinstated. Nostalgia
also operates on more localised levels as evidenced in fan movements to
save threatened sports teams or in promoted conservative boundaries
around community as lived through support of a sporting team as Gary
Robson demonstrates in his case study of English football club Millwall
and its supporters (Robson, 2000).

Sporting traditions are made and perpetuated in several ways, however. They are formed through lived and shared experiences, but are also
mediated through, newspapers, popular periodicals, television and radio,
books for the popular market written by journalists and sport historians
and the work of academic sport historians. All of these groups construct,
reconstruct and even invent interpretations of sporting events that are
then digested by the wider public and by political, economic and cultural
elites. Sporting traditions are then presented to the public in a variety of
ways as part of its collective experience as members of a particular region
or nation. This is done to sell particular philosophies, products and political policies.

In the English-speaking world in particular, sport has been equated
with masculinity – real men play and watch sport, especially the dominant team sports of a football code in winter and either cricket or baseball in summer. As a result, there has been little room for women in nostalgic reminiscences of sport unless they conjure up images of acceptable
femininity like Helen Wills Moody, Chris Evert or a host of successful
figure skaters in the American case. In a powerful analysis of sport in
American society, Mariah Burton Nelson (1994) states that "the stronger
women get, the more men love football". Thus as women enter into an
increasing variety of sports and achieve success, nostalgia in the sporting
realm takes on a particular gendered force. As such, while this discussion
focuses on "national" and "club" levels for the most part, it is clear that

while not limited to men, sporting nostalgia is a heavily gendered phenomenon.

In New Zealand, Australia and South Africa (among whites) nostalgic representations of past sporting successes and heroes have been closely linked with a nostalgia for a simpler past when everyone knew their place and real men played football (be it in rugby union, rugby league or Australian football). Rapid social, economic and political changes in these countries (although these have been much more pronounced in South Africa) have led many to focus on the simpler days of the past. In New Zealand during the 1990s, nostalgia centred on the 1956 rugby tour by the South Africans as the last time the country was "truly united" before protests movements of the 1960s-80s and the rationalist economic policies of 1984 and beyond.

While sports history in the United States has progressed further than in many countries, the production and use of sports history has not escaped myth and some distortions of focus. Americans are constantly bombarded with images from their sporting past that are used to promote American ideals and consumerism in the present. No sport has been more infused with nostalgic meaning than American baseball.

Case Study 1: The USA

Baseball, so the mythical version goes, began when Abner Doubleday organised a game in 1839 in Cooperstown, a small town in a farming area of upstate New York. As we know, in reality, baseball emerged from English ball games and developed in the urban cities of the northeastern United States. Clubs were formed in New York and other cities from the 1840s. Thus, what developed as an urban adaptation has been mythologised as a rural and uniquely American game, in part, to cover up its roots in an English game played primarily by girls and also to provide a history that ties baseball to an idealised (or a later Norman Rockwellised) version of the American past. Certainly, sport historians of the latter twentieth century have not deliberately perpetuated the foundation myth of baseball, but it is still widely believed within American society. Other myths about baseball as the essence of American culture and identity have appeared which, nevertheless, establish a form of mystical aura around the game.

American movies of the 1980s, 1990s and beyond such as *The Natural, Eight Men Out, Field of Dreams, The Babe, 61* and *For the Love of the Game* rekindled baseball's nostalgic presentation through the use of real and mythical images. The symbolic setting of "Field of Dreams" on a farm in the American "heartland" of Iowa perfectly demonstrates the links between baseball, pastoralism and the essence of Americanness. When Shoeless Joe Jackson asks Ray Kinsella "Is this heaven?" and the answer is

"No, it's Iowa," American audiences can easily make the links between the two as Iowa has been presented as the "heartland," indeed, the essence of an idealised, pastoral America. In addition, these films collectively represent a version of the American and baseballing past that are dominated by white males, although women have been represented in the film version of their baseball past in *A League of Their Own.*

Why is baseball significant? Baseball lost its former pre-eminence as America's national pastime as football and later basketball increased their fan support during the television age. For many a more alarming development was that by the 1980s, more American children were playing soccer than Little League baseball. It should be no surprise that baseball movies, Ronald Reagan, the most nostalgic of American Presidents, and the preponderance of sport history work on baseball all appeared by the early 1980s. By the end of the 1970s, many Americans felt that the country had been drifting since the assassination of John Kennedy in 1963. Failure in Vietnam, the end of official segregation, the rise of rock-and-roll music, the increasing use of drugs, urban decay and the shift in immigration from white-dominated to Latin American and Asian countries all combined to create a tremendous sense of insecurity among white middle class and middle aged Americans in the 1970s and 1980s. Not surprisingly, this led to the appearance of groups such as the Moral Majority (though always a minority in reality) and a resurgent and nostalgic conservatism embodied in President Reagan. Reagan took images of the American past and even those of the present, including those from sport, in developing a sense of longing for a return to "traditional American values" which shaped a once great past. Indeed, Reagan was personally connected to an idealised sporting past through his own portrayal of famed Notre Dame player George Gipp in the film *Knute Rockne: All-American.* On his deathbed Gipp/Reagan asked coach Rockne to have the boys "win one for the Gipper", a phrase that became a prime motivating force in American sport and one of the most recognised statements in US public discourse.

While not directly serving the interests of political groups or their uses of nostalgic images, sport historians working in the United States have contributed to nostalgic representations of the American sporting past. In examining the number of books published by sport historians in the United States, or in looking at the papers presented at annual sports history conferences, one cannot help but notice an overwhelming focus on baseball. While baseball has been the most important sport in American society at certain times of the past, the amount of study devoted to baseball remains striking. Unlike countries with small academic communities like New Zealand or South Africa, the reason cannot be attributed to a paucity of scholars in the field, so answers must be sought elsewhere.

The production of sports history in the 1970s and 1980s cannot be divorced from the wider trends in American society. Given the threats to baseball as the dominant American sport in the present, one way to shore up its position is through appeals to the past. Books like David Voigt's *America Through Baseball* (1976) appealed for readers to view baseball as a central element in American history and society. For Voigt, baseball has mirrored American society since the mid-nineteenth century. Other scholars do not focus quite as specifically on the notion of "mirroring" but suggest that American history and identity can be "read" through baseball and baseball history. As a result, much of academic baseball history would agree with the statements by fictional character Terence Mann (played by James Earle Jones) in *Field of Dreams* when he states that baseball has marked the time in American society and has ruled it "like an army of steamrollers" or that the one constant in American society has always been baseball. While baseball cannot be ignored as an important element in the history of American popular culture, there is not enough critical analysis of the production of baseball's position, both independent of and in relation to other sports, or on baseball's historical role in excluding women and African-Americans while providing an inclusive identity for white males. If baseball is the essence of Americanness, then it has largely been a white, male Americanness for much of its history.

Baseball remains firmly tied to a cultural nostalgic paradigm pervading American middle class society in the 1990s and beyond, particularly after the spectacular home run records set by Mark Maguire, Sammy Sosa and Barry Bonds in the late 1990s and early 2000s. The tenacity of nostalgic views of baseball was demonstrated in a 1991 article by Ronald Story which was also been reprinted in the 1995 David Wiggins edited volume *Sport in America: From Wicked Amusement to National Obsession*. Story begins by stating:

> We know we love it [baseball] above all others. But why do we? Or rather, since it started a long time ago, why *did* we? Why *baseball* and not some other sport? Or *no* sport? And why baseball with such passionate single-mindedness rather than as one sport among many? How did this come to be? (Story, 1995: 121).

Aside from the broad assumptions that are virtually impossible to substantiate, Story's opening still suggests some essentialist form for baseball as central to American character. He goes on to suggest that baseball became popular in the 1880s because men loved it since they played it when they were young. Story concludes by stating that the country was in turmoil in the 1860s and 1870s and baseball embodied security and control, comradeship and recognition and spread these throughout the country. "Because adolescent boys of that generation needed them, baseball became their salvation and their love. And they never forgot it. In partial payment, they made it the American game" (Story, 1995: 132). While Story is to be commended for searching for the historical moment when baseball became the "national game" in the States, he further entrenches nostalgia within the history of baseball through the general linking of youth culture and baseball while leaving much unsubstantiated. Story is not alone as other recent accounts also view baseball in a nostalgic light such as Richard Skolink's 1994 book, *Baseball and the Pursuit of Innocence*. Whether baseball is conceptualised as some sort of historical "mirror" of American society or seen as the "essence" or "expression" of Americanness, nostalgia pervades analysis and the presentation of baseball and much sport history in general, especially when contextualised with broader nostalgic impulses in American culture and politics of the 1980s and 1990s. Recent books examining the creation of American football as a mass American spectacle such as Michael Oriard's *Reading Football* (1993) and *King Football* (2001) have begun to provide a greater corrective to the concentration on baseball within American male sport history and also point to fruitful lines of analysis through examination of media representation in establishing a prominent position for dominant sports. Even beyond this additional research, one could easily argue that football has been more pervasive within American culture in the past few decades, especially after reading accounts like Harold Bissinger's (1991) in *Friday Night Lights*.

The United States provides an extreme case for many examples of social issues affecting first world or Western societies, but the problems of immigration, changing economic realities and greater global ties are certainly not unique to the USA. A similar reading of Margaret Thatcher and John Major's Britain demonstrates that Reagan did not have a monopoly on representing a nostalgic past in the face of present social, political and moral crises. In addition, once relatively isolated societies like New Zealand and Australia have also faced these "crises" of immigration, globalisation and economic restructuring. New Zealand provides a useful additional example to the American case in illustrating the operation of nostalgia in sport.

Case Study 2: New Zealand

In New Zealand, nostalgic representations of rugby attempt to take people back to the days before the violence of the 1981 South African tour and to a time when New Zealanders seemed more united, as they appeared to be during the 1956 South African tour. Nostalgia for the New Zealand of the 1950s, when the country briefly led the world in standard of living, emerged alongside a rationalist economic discourse that threatens to divide New Zealanders further as it also promoted economic growth and free trade as the new path to national prosperity.

While the government pursued new policies (with both major parties following a neo-liberal economic rationalist agenda), it and the media also promoted a New Zealand national identity that clung to past masculine glories in sports (particularly rugby) and war. Advertisers increasingly have used rugby to advertise their products now that the sport appeared to have been de-politicised with the end of South African isolation. An excellent example of this has been the Bank of New Zealand's 1992 and 1993 television advertising campaign "Who are you? You're a New Zealander, and who are we? We're your bank". Their commercial shows the Hokianga rugby ground with its arch of remembrance for the fallen soldiers of the world wars, thus closely and symbolically linking the two most powerful cultural symbols of New Zealand masculinist national identity.

Much writing on sports history by journalists and academics have also fit into the nostalgic representation of New Zealand society and history (Barrow, 1992; Crawford, 1986; Roger, 1991; Zavos, 1997), though such writings have been subjected to critical review (MacLean, 1997; Nauright, 1994). Most sports history writings in New Zealand discuss rugby, which is consistently presented as the "national game". Despite such assertions, the experiences of Maori, Pacific Islander or female rugby players are rarely presented as central, though after losing in the semifinal of the 1999 Rugby World Cup and losing in the Tri-Nations series with Australia and South Africa and the Bledisloe Cup to Australia, the only international champions and cup holders in 2000 were the "Black Ferns" the national women's rugby team.

Rugby came under attack in the 1970s and 1980s, particularly over New Zealand's links with South Africa (Black & Nauright, 1998; Nauright & Black, 1996). During the 1981 tour of South Africa to New Zealand, women's groups assailed rugby for increasing their domestic labour (Thompson, 1988) while Maori groups protested against the focus on racism in South Africa while racism also was prevalent in New Zealand. The violent response of the government and police to the tactics of protestors led many to question the values that had brought New Zealand to such a point. As a result, many parents withdrew their sons from rugby and encouraged them to participate in other sports such as soccer. The 1981 tour created a moment of hegemonic crisis as threats to the established order of a white-male and rugby dominated New Zealand came to the fore. The threat to rugby was compounded by New Zealand's qualification for the 1982 soccer World Cup Finals that greatly heightened the popular images for its increasing share of younger sports participants.

As a result of this "crisis", new initiatives were taken in the late 1980s and early 1990s to involve more children in rugby. Modified games and a new marketing image appeared and rugby began to recover, particularly as New Zealand won the inaugural Rugby World Cup held in Australia and New Zealand in 1987. Positive advertising in the early 1990s and the promotion of fair and clean play in youth rugby further aided in the renewed popularity of rugby. Despite its media portrayal as a game embodying the essence of New Zealandness and a game with a new, improved and "cleaner" image, rugby remains as a cultural form that promotes violence, the denigration of women and homosexuals and is built on the backs of women's domestic service (Thompson, 1988; 1990).

Professional and amateur historians of New Zealand sport have contributed to the almost exclusive national focus on rugby through the generation of dozens of histories of rugby. Academic analysis has been imbued with nostalgic reflection on occasion (Crawford, 1986) or inaccuracies that promote a rural mythology (Phillips, 1987). Indeed, the prevailing sociological analysis of rugby up to the 1990s was on its role as a "secular religion" (Crawford, 1986) and even as "the very corner-stone of society" (Cleveland, 1966; Crawford, 1978). While such interpretations are correct in delineating rugby's powerful place in New Zealand popular culture, they have become virtual clichés that have obscured other possible analyses. Rugby has not always been a unifying force for all New Zealanders – such as generations of women who have provided domestic servicing for rugby or the thousands of New Zealanders who supported rugby boycotts against South Africa while the apartheid regime held power there. These groups have been excluded and even denigrated by the rugby culture.

In the restructured New Zealand social arena, protests against playing South Africa in rugby are too often characterised as merely a short-term aberration and an inconvenience caused by a few well-organised radicals (Barrow, 1992). The danger is that such a view is already dominant in New Zealand where rugby and the rugby culture, with tremendous help from the New Zealand media and big business, have regained their positions that suffered so much in the aftermath of 1981. Rather than seeking to draw on the diversity of opinions in New Zealand, the old white male cultural hegemony has been maintained and repackaged for popular consumption. Conservative elements also promote old, tough rugby heroes as models of what a true "kiwi bloke" should be like. The stereotypical hero is embodied in Colin Meads, hero of 1960s All Black teams. Meads grew up in a sheep-farming region and went on to be one of the greatest forwards in the game. He represents the essence of conservative New Zealand's ideal man – a sheep farming, successful rugby player. In reality, the majority of All Black representatives have come from professional occupations and major urban centres (Ryan, 2001).

Prospects for future political and cultural challenges to white male and middle class hegemony may even be more difficult than in the past. It is not likely that a social issue dealing with international cultural contacts will emerge in the near future to so divide the soul of New Zealand society. With the support of big business and television, a repackaged rugby may also be harder to attack. Renewed focus on national symbols and national identity in the wake of the 1990 celebrations of 150 years since the signing of the Treaty of Waitangi, which incorporated Maoris in the wider legal society at least, have reinforced dominant values. One of the most potent symbols is that of the silver fern worn by New Zealand sporting teams and especially the silver fern incorporated on the jerseys of the "All Blacks", the national rugby team. Cleveland referred to the All Black jersey itself as a symbol identifying the team that represents the country (Cleveland, 1967). The All Black jersey can even be worn nostalgically as the Canterbury Company markets old styles of All Black jerseys, particularly that worn by the 1905 "Original" All Blacks. This process is similar to the marketing of baseball nostalgia apparel and "vintage" football (soccer) jerseys in England.

Recent works on rugby attest to its power in New Zealand popular culture They also demonstrate the ways in which nostalgia and sports history, be it academic or journalistic, reinforce male (largely white and middle class) hegemony and can serve to create new forms of cultural conservatism that hearken back to the glory days of old. The New Zealand case shows how hegemonic cultural values can be used to underpin economic changes and to marginalise protests by feminists, ecologists and other groups. The old order has been restored in a concrete sense through the return of international rugby matches with arch-rival South Africa in 1992, a South African tour of New Zealand in 1994 and the 1995 Rugby World Cup final being contested by the two nations, though the onset of professionalism and the prominence of 1991 and 1999 Rugby World Cup champions, Australia, has altered the international rugby hierarchy and advanced trans-Tasman rivalry since 1995. The rapid expansion of media driven global corporatism in sport during the 1990s (though the process began earlier) fundamentally altered sporting structures as tensions emerged between identity and nostalgia in sport as lived experience and a new media-driven nostalgia centred on brand loyalty, consumerism and individual sporting celebrities.

Fans, Nostalgia and Sport as a Capitalist Enterprise

I have discussed elsewhere the dramatic changes that have occurred within modern achievement sport practice in the past couple of decades (Nauright et al, 2003). Sports and sporting events have become increasingly central in a global political economy that has seen production shift from developed to less developed societies with an ever expanding focus on 'branding', 'theming' and consumption of image and lifestyle (see Gottdiener, 2001; Klein, 2001). From the restyling of large-scale sports events as entertainment extravaganzas, sports events have become mega-entertainment leisure and tourist events as sport competes with other forms of entertainment in the marketplace, for television contracts and sponsorships. This process has a long history in North America while in Europe and other parts of the world it is a more recent phenomenon. In the late 1980s, in 'Blueprint for the Future of Football', the Football Association in England promoted the conversion of 'going to a match' on a Saturday into having 'integrated leisure experiences' (quoted in Taylor, 1992: 192). In this process, it is hoped that, in the style of North American sport, football matches would attract fans to a festive family atmosphere in opposition to its hooligan image. Following on from the transformation of sports matches into leisure events, sporting and other events have become central parts of urban economic and regional and national tourism development strategies.

In this context the 'essence' of sport may be shifting as sport moves ever further towards being fully enmeshed in a global sport-media-tourism nexus where sports events are viewed as integral parts of local, regional and national development strategies and as sports become more fully integrated with multinational corporations such as Nike and Adidas, and media conglomerates such as Rupert Murdoch's web of companies. It is clear that there is increasing control over the operation of sport and sporting competitions by major national and international media outlets, but there has also been resistance to the changes brought on by ever increasing scale and globalisation of competitions.

In this process traditional sports fans, local communities and democratic practices often are discarded or ignored as the philosophy of growth is promoted and business and governments align in support of events driven economies (see for example Rosentraub, 1999). The end result, in English soccer, for example, was an increase in pricing for match tickets at the lowest end from £2-£4 for a standing place in the early 1980s at English First Division matches, to around £25-£30 per ticket on average for the cheapest seats for Premier League matches in the English Premier League in 2001-2. The rise in costs for match attendance has put significant strains on the ability of working class men, football's historic primary constituent, to afford to maintain their traditional spectating habits and indeed those who have been able to do so, have seen much of their disposable income diverted into their football support. Pay television operators and clubs realised this and moved to capitalise by attempting to convert many to virtual supporting practices. Indeed, during the 2001-2 season, SKY television offered special television pay-per-view packages for Premier League matches at £8-£12, well in excess of the 1980s cost for live attendance. As a result, many of the traditional supporters of football have been forced into virtual spectatorship either of live matches on pay tv outlets SKY and ITV Sports or await the limited highlight packages on free-to-air channels.

In the process of fully commodifying their product and turning supporters into consumers of the team's brand, Football clubs in England took steps to diversify their product and sell a wide range of leisure and entertainment activities and financial services to their supporters (Nauright et al 2002). While e-branding is becoming common, it is not a one way street and cyberspace has also enabled supporter associations and other groups to mobilise support for clubs under threat (Nauright et al 2002) Supporter campaigns do have some success in mobilising support against mergers and relocations (Phillips et al, 2002; Phillips & Nauright, 1999), however, the main structures of the media-sport complex have emerged largely unscathed as large-scale sport progresses from localised social and community events, to globalised mediated ones. As a result, sport has emerged more fully integrated into a new global political economy as part of a sport-media-tourism complex (Nauright et al, 2003) that privileges the global over the local in the service of new strategies of capitalist accumulation.

Conclusion

Structurally, sport has changed in recent times, though its power in generating lasting memories that are vital parts of the human experience can be utilised to promote wider identifications, consumption and loyalty. In times of rapid social, cultural, political and economic change, sport is a constant that, while evolving and changing itself, remains recognisable and retains cultural currency often reminding fans of "all that once was good, and could be again" (*Field of Dreams*). *Field of Dreams* was prophetic in claiming that "people will come" to Iowa to see the old baseball players restored to their former glory as thousands flock to the field to play catch or take a turn at bat. Fathers take their sons to football matches throughout the world in attempts to transfer their team identification across the generations. Thus, while sport and sporting nostalgia is used for broader political and economic purposes, sport retains a powerful cultural essence that is a fundamental marker of identity in the modern era.

References

Barrow, G. (1992). *All Blacks versus Springboks: A Century of Rugby Rivalry*. Auckland: Reed Books.

Bateman, A. (2002). "More mighty than the bat, the pen . . .": Culture, Hegemony and the Literaturisation of cricket. Paper presented to the British Society for Sports History Annual Conference, Leicester, 13 April.

Bissinger, H. (1991). *Friday Night Lights: A Town, a Team, and a Dream*. New York: Harper Perennial, 1991.

Black, D. & Nauright, J. (1998). *Rugby and the South African Nation*. Manchester: Manchester University Press.

Cleveland, L. (1966). Political Football: The Role of Rugby and the Press in New Zealand political culture. *Comment*, June, 23-30.

Cleveland, L. (1967). Pop art, Politics and Sport in New Zealand. *Politics*, 1(2), 200-215.

Connerton, P. (1988). *How Societies Remember*. Cambridge: Cambridge University Press.

Crawford, S. (1978). New Zealand Rugby: Vigorous, Violent and Vicious? *Review of Sport and Leisure*, 3(1), 64-83.

Crawford, S. (1986). A Secular Religion: The Historical Iconography of New Zealand Rugby. *Physical Education Review*, 8(2), 146-158.

DaSilva, F. & Faught, J. (1982). Nostalgia: A Sphere and Process of Contemporary Ideology. *Qualitative Sociology*, 5(1).

Davis, F. (1979). *Yearning for Yesterday: A Sociology of Nostalgia*. New York: The Fress Press.

Giamatti, A.B. (1989). *Take Time for Paradise: Americans and their Games*. New York: Simon & Schuster.

Goksøyr, M. (1998). Football, Development and Identity in a Small Nation: Football, Culture, Spectators and Playing Styles in Twentieth Century Norway. *Football Studies*, 1(1), 37-47.

Gottdiener, M. (2001). The theming of America: American Dreams, Media Fantasies, and Themed Environments. 2nd Edition. Boulder: Westview.

Gruneau, R. (1983). *Class, Sports and Social Development*. Amherst: University of Massachusetts Press.

Gruneau, R. (1993). Critique of Sport in Modernity: Theorising Power, Culture and the Politics of the Body (pp. 85-109). In E.Dunning, J. Maguire & R. Pearton (eds), *The Sports Process*. Champaign: Human Kinetics.

Hargreaves, J. (1986). *Sport, Power and Culture*. Cambridge: Polity Press.

Hornby, N. (2000). *Fever Pitch*. New edition. London: Penguin.

Ingham, A.G. & Loy, J.W. (eds) (1993). *Sport in Social Development: Traditions, Transitions and transformations*. Champaign: Human Kinetics, 1993.

Klein, N. (2001). *No Logo*. London: Flamingo.

Lipsyte, R. (1975). *Sportsworld: An American Dreamland*. New York: Quadrangle/ New York Times.

Lowenthal, D. (1985). *The Past is a Foreign Country*. Cambridge: Cambridge

MacLean, M. (1997). Some Hope in Rugby Writing, but the Blokes are still in Control. *Sporting Traditions*, 14(1), 135-145.

Maguire, J. (1999). *Global sport: Identities, Societies, Civilizations*. Cambridge: Polity.

Nauright, J. (1994). Reclaiming Old and Forgotten Heroes: Nostalgia, Rugby and Identity in New Zealand. *Sporting Traditions*, 10(2), 131-139.

Nauright, J. & Black, D. (1996). Hitting Them Where it Hurts: Springbok – All Black Rugby, Masculine National Identity and Counter-hegemonic Struggle, 1959-1992. In J. Nauright & T.J.L. Chandler (eds), *Making Men: Rugby and Masculine Identity* (pp. 205-226). London: Frank Cass.

Nauright, J., Garcia, B. & Miah, A. (2002). The International Political Economy of Sport in the Twenty-first Century. In J. Nauright & K. Schimmel (eds), *The Political Economy of Sport* (in press). Basingstoke: Palgrave.

Nelson, M.B. (1994). *The Stronger Women get, the More Men Love Football*. New York: Harcourt Brace.

Novak, M. (1993/1976). *The Joy of Sports*. Madison: Madison Books.

Oriard, M. (1993). *Reading Football: How the Popular Press Created a National Spectacle*. Chapel Hill: University of North Carolina Press.

Oriard, M. (2001). *King Football*. Chapel Hill: University of North Carolina Press.

Phillips, J.O.C. (1987). *A Man's Country: The Image of the Pakeha Male*. Auckland: Penguin.

Phillips, M.G., Hutchins, B. & Stewart, B. (2002). The Media Sport Cultural Complex: Football and Fan Resistance in Australia. In In J. Nauright & K. Schimmel (eds), *The Political Economy of Sport* (in press). Basingstoke: Palgrave.

Phillips, M.G. & Nauright, J. 1999. Fan Movements to Save Teams Threatened with Amalgamation in Different Football Codes in Australia. *International Sports Studies*, 17(1), 23-38.

Robson, G. (2000). *No one Likes Us, We don't Care: The myth and Reality of Millwall Fandom*. Oxford: Berg.

Roger, W. (1991). *Old Heroes: The 1956 Springbok Tour and the Lives Beyond*. Auckland: Hodder & Stoughton.

Rosentraub, M. (1999). Major League Losers: The Real Cost of Sports and who's Paying for it. Revised edition. New York: Basic Books.

Ryan, G. (2001). Rural Myth and Urban Actuality: The Anatomy of All Black and New Zealand Rugby 1884-1938. *New Zealand Journal of History*, 35(1).

Skolink, R. (1994). *Baseball and the Pursuit of Innocence*. College Station: Texas A&M University Press, 1994.

Springwood, C.F. (1996). *From Cooperstown to Dyresville: A Geography of Baseball Nostalgia*. Boulder: Westview.

Stewart, K (1988). Nostalgia – a Polemic. *Cultural Anthropology*, 3(3).

Story, R. (1995). The Country of the Young: The Meaning of Baseball in Early American Culture. In D. Wiggins (ed.), *Sport in America: From Wicked Amusement to National Obsession*. Champaign: Human Kinetics.

Taylor, R. (1992). *Football and its Fans: Supporters and their Relation with the Game, 1885-1985*. Leicester: Leicester University Press.

Thompson, S. (1988). Challenging the hegemony: New Zealand Women's Opposition to Rugby. *International Review for the Sociology of Sport*, 23, 205-212.

Thompson, S. (1990). "Thank the Ladies for the Plates": The Incorporation of Women into Sport. *Leisure Studies*, 9, 135-143.

Voigt, D.Q. (1976) *America Through Baseball*. New York: Burnham Inc.

Zavos, S. (1997). *Winters of Revenge*. Auckland: Penguin.

Three Dimensions of Playing the Game: About Mouth Pull, Tug-of-War and Sportization

Henning Eichberg

Scene: Two human beings are standing shoulder to shoulder. They put their arms around their partners' necks, mutually, symmetrically, like good friends. Opening their lips, each inserts a forefinger into the other's mouth. And then, at a signal, they begin to pull. Their mouths and cheeks become distorted, their eyes roll, their faces assume grotesque expressions. The competitors tug and tug. Intensifying their efforts, they turn their heads outward, trying to relieve their pain and to resist effectively. Finally, one of them will give up, at first slowly, following the pull by turning his head and then overtly surrendering by turning the rest of his body. He is defeated.

If sport has no 'essence' – then what?

What is sport, what is its essence? People have posed this question for generations, and this symposium has raised this question anew. At the same time, this question confronts a fundamental problem. Sport is regarded as a specifically modern form of culture which assumes specific patterns in space and time, showing characteristic configurations of social interaction, cultural energy and social meaning – but having no *"Wesen"*, no essence of the universal type which the pedagogues of physical education and ideologists of Olympic sport have tried to define. The discourse of *Wesen*, the construction of a universally human "essence" and its associated concept of "function" – may even hinder an understanding of sport, just as essentialism in general rather hinders the understanding of other cultural phenomena. The notion of the essential must be dealt with by means of cultural critique.

If not epistemologically convincing in itself, the question of essence may, nevertheless, have an empirical meaning. It is not by accident that it rises from time to time in certain societal situations – not unlike the question of "God". The question expresses a crucial crisis within the cultural sphere. Today it is doping that provides new reasons to challenge ideas about the *Wesen* of sport (Møller 1999). Does sport belong to the field of ethics or aesthetics – is it a school of morals or a kind of art – or something else? That is why questions about essentialism deserve answers, even if we do not accept the authority of essentialism as a doctrine. If we want to avoid the trap of a reified *Wesen*, we can ask questions from the other direction – by looking at what is *not* sport. One way to do this is to look more closely at a physical activity like the mouth pull.

An Inuit game ...

The Inuit game of mouth pull is not a sport in the modern sense. There is no Olympic discipline of mouth pulling, nor in all likelihood will there ever be one. But is it, perhaps, a sport, nonetheless? And if it is not, why might mouth pulling be misunderstood as being a sport? Indeed, other Inuit games and activities like "Eskimo boxing," along with pull-and-tug competitions that occur in other non-Western cultures, have typically been categorized as "sport" by sports anthropologists (Larsen 1972, Ulf 1981, Howell 1996). In a similar vein, sports historians have presented popular Old European pastimes like *Fingerhakeln*, finger pulling, as early forms of "sport".

At first glance, mouth pulling will appear as physical action that is competitive and oriented towards performance. Since it includes these three elements, the mouth tug fulfils the basic criteria for sport as they have been proposed in sociological analyses that define sport in terms of bodily action, competition and performance (Tangen 1997, 38-40). On the other hand, one might have certain doubts: Is tug-the-mouth really sport? These doubts are reinforced when we take a closer look at the cultural context of the game.

The mouth pull was practised in the traditional world of the Inuit, the Arctic Eskimo. During the long, dark winter season, when the sun remains below the horizon for months at a time, people draw closer to each other in their communal long houses where every family has a sort of cell with a sleeping bench and an oil lamp. In the dancing houses, or *kashim*, the drums are pounding during a state of permanent festivity. The drum dance, the *ingmerneq* or *qilaatersorneq*, makes people high and provokes them to laughter. The shamans, or *angákoq*, practice their ecstatic healing rituals, causing their companions to enter into states of altered consciousness. In this atmosphere of social warmth and intensity, it happens that people challenge each other, and especially the strong men. Besides fisticuffs and competitions that involve lifting and balancing, a lot of pull-and-tug games are practised: to tug the stick (*arsâraq* or *quertemilik*) or the match stick; to pull the rope (*norqutit*) or the smooth seal skin (*asârniûneq*); the arm pull; the finger, wrist or hand pull; the neck, ear or foot pull; the elbow pull (*pakásungmingneq*); and wrist pressing *(mûmigtut)*. For competitive pleasure, people may tug or twist each other's noses or ears – or, among the men, even the testicles (Mauss 1904/05; Jensen 1965; Joelsen in: Idrætten 1978; Keewatin 1989, 31-42).

During the summer, the traditional Inuit society changed its social character in fundamental ways. It dissolved into nuclear families, forming smaller groups of hunters and collectors. They met again, however, at summer festivals, or *aasivik*, where drum dances and competitions again played a central role. One of these summer events was rendered on canvas by the famous Greenlandic painter Aron of Kangeq (1822-1869), showing one of the most eccentric pulling exercises – pulling arse. In an open-air scene, one sees a group of ten Inuit assembled around two men competing with their trousers pulled down. Jens Kreutzmann (1828-1899), a collector of popular stories and traditions, described in greater detail how people used for this purpose a short rope with two pieces of wood fastened at the ends. They put these pieces into their backsides so they could tug the rope by using their back muscles (Thisted 1997, 152-154).

... and other cultures of pull and tug

From other societies, tug-and-pull games are known that may look similar to, though less eccentric than, these Inuit games (Grundfeld 1975, 206-207; Endrei/Zolnay 1986, 92-93, XIV). We know pulling competitions especially from ancient Scandinavia (Bjarnason 1905, 134-141; Steijskal 1954, 54-65, 141-44, 164-66; Wahlqvist 1979, 125-27; Møller 1990/91, 4, 14-35; Hellspong 2000a, 101-2), from Celtic cultures (F'loch/Peru 1987, 9-16; Novacek 1989, 43, 71; Jarvie 1991) as well as from the Pacific, from Melanesian and Polynesian societies, and from Africa (Ulf 1981, 25; Howell 1996, 1087, 1090).

The multiplicity of forms includes simple actions involving finger, arm and neck pulling, tug-of-war and stick pulling, along with more complex variations like the Danish game "To pull the calf from the cow" *(Rykke kalven fra koen)*. In "To tie up the peewit" *(Snøre vibe)*, the opponents try to topple each other by means of a rope connecting their feet. In "To cut out Palle's eye" *(Stikke Palles øje ud)*, the two competitors try – backside to backside and not unlike the Inuit arse tug – to pull a stick between their legs towards a candle which they try to extinguish. So-called hide games, Old Nordic *skinnleikr*, were different variations on pulling hide or skin, which could resemble ball games, but could also develop towards the belt pull (Old Nordic *beltadráttr*) and rope pull *(reipdráttr)*. A Nordic variation of the latter was "ring pull", *at toga honk*, where two men, normally in a sitting position, pulled a rope that formed a ring. In the form of the "four men's pull" this could also become a group game where each of the pullers tried to reach a certain object, while the others prevented this from happening by their tricky rhythmic pulls, trying at the same time to reach their own respective objects.

The pulling games were often connected with joking, so that the physical action exploded into shared laughter. So when reconstructing the socio-cultural climate of Inuit mouth pull, one should imagine, instead of a sports hall, a smoky pub somewhere in the Alps where strong men, laughing and drinking beer, challenge each other to *Fingerhakeln*, in the era before finger pulling became an element of modern Bavarian folklore.

The parallels between these popular cultures of pull and tug should, however, not be overemphasized. The medieval Danish historian Saxo Grammaticus told of the Danish king Erik Ejegod, who liked tug-of-war and practised it so often that he was able, while sitting, to pull, with one rope in each hand, four men towards himself. We may assume that this amused those people, but the activity was not always as harmless. Another man, Erik Målspage, pulled the rope in a competition with a lord Vestmar, both men having wagered their lives. When Erik finally won after a hard fight – "*exerting his full strength by means of both hands and feet*", as Saxo described it – he neither dismissed the loser with noble "sporting" generosity, nor did the competition dissolve into laughter in the Inuit manner. Erik put his foot on the back of his opponent, breaking his backbone and, to be quite sure of his victory, broke his neck, too, accompanying this with insulting words (Wahlqvist 1979, 125-6).

Whether we believe these stories or not, and however representative they may or may not have been, they bear witness to a warrior culture which placed brutal pull-and-tug games in the context of competing and killing (Eichberg 1983, 1990). This was dramatically different both from the sociability of the Inuit winter house, from Bavarian folklore and from the modern sport of tug-of-war. Yet tug-of-war is not an unambiguous modern sport, either. Though much less eccentric than mouth pull, tug-of-war encountered some problems that have denied it recognition as an Olympic sport.

As it moved in the direction of modern sport, the tug-of-war passed through the Scottish Highland Games. When these games were resumed in 1819, after a period during which they were suppressed by the English, they included piping, dancing, foot races and stone lifting. Already in 1822, however, it was reported that "*the most remarkable feature was the tearing of three cows limb from limb after they had been felled*" (Novak 1989, 43). It is not documented that this was a direct continuation of traditions from older Highland Games. In fact, the feud culture of the Scottish clan society was characterized by cattle raids, which were directed against the property of other clans (Jarvie 1991, 27). It is not impossible that this practise was transferred to games like pull-the-cow. In the early nineteenth century, however, with Sir Walter Scott's imaginary version of the "wild" Highland Scots, it could also be romanticized and the game of tug-of-cow thus be "invented" as folklore, displaying an entertaining look at an imagined barbarism.

Whether the game of tug was an artificial romantic construction or had its roots in older practices remains an open question. In any case, it was starting in the 1840s that tug-of-war appeared on the programs of various Scottish Highland Games and soon became a specific feature – side by side with tossing the caber – of their particular athletic culture (Jarvie 1991, cover illustration). In the Scottish Highland Games that were held in Paris in 1889, the combination of tug-of-war, caber tossing, Highland dancing and tartan fashion already resembled an ethno-pop show, organized as it was side by side with Buffalo Bill's Wild West Show (Novak 1989, 71).

During the early phase of modern sport, this Scottish game of tug existed along with popular traditions in English villages and towns. At the London market place, rope pull was held annually on Shrove Tuesday. It was said that up to 2000 people participated in the tug event and held a festival afterwards where the rope was sold. The custom was regarded as dating back to the time of King Henry VI and connected with the fight between a red and a white party, or the War of the Roses, one side fighting for the king and the other for the Duke of York (Georgens 1883, 155).

In a similar fashion, from the late eighteenth century onwards, philanthropical educationalists on the European continent rediscovered the popular tugging games. They integrated pull and tug, often in an abstract and systematic way, into their handbooks of exercises, gymnastics and games, adding health-related and moralistic recommendations (Guts Muths 1793, 356-358; also Hvormed 1861, 1). In spite of this pedagogization, pulling games were often "overlooked" in the gymnastic literature of the nineteenth century, until tug-of-war reappeared as sport at the end of the century (detailed table in: Møller 1996, 11).

As a competitive sport, tug-of-war was adopted around 1880 by the Amateur Athletic Association (AAA) in England and seemed by the beginning of twentieth century to be on its way to being established as an Olympic discipline. However, it was soon excluded from the Olympic canon, since it was regarded by serious athletes "*as something of a joke*" (Arlott 1975, 1058). Since 1958 the Tug of War International Federation (TWIF) has been working on a regular system of champion-ships with weight classes and detailed rules for their competitions. Recently, observers expected that tug-of-war would soon return to the Olympic programme (James 2000, 402).

The exclusion of tug-of-war from Olympic sport is, from an analytical standpoint, at least as interesting as its reverse, the modern integration of the game into sport. Historically, rope-pulling competitions took their place somewhere between the eccentricity of mouth pull (or even arse pull) and the rationality of modern sport. There is something "unserious" in tug-of-war, too, and this opens the door to the key question of what *does* constitutes the "serious" element in sport.

The quest for categories and contradictions

Not only must we ask questions about the classification of tug-of-war as a sport, we can also take the analysis one step further: Which type of sport? When we categorize mouth tug under the rubric of "pull" – side by side with finger-pull and tug-of-war – even this classification is not self-evident, nor is it as unproblematical, as one might think at first glance. It calls for associations that seem, socio-culturally, too "natural": in that pull is, along with other "natural" or "elementary" activities like running, jumping, throwing and lifting, a competition of man-against-man, an attempt to triumph over another person, to beat him (and it is nearly always him, not her), to defeat him, to overcome the other, and that this victory has "by nature" a positive value. In the analytical literature, the games of pull and tug are normally and self-evidently categorized as belonging to the genre of competition and fighting. On the basis of this assumption, one scholar has used categories like "*games and trials of strength (lifting weights, pulling games)*" (Dufaitre 1989, 6), in German *Zieh- und Schiebekämpfe* (Ulf 1981, 25-26), in French *jeux athletiques/jeux de force* (Floc'h/Peru 1987) and in Danish *kamp- og kaplege* (games of fight and competition, Møller 1990/91, vol.4). However, does the Inuit game of mouth pull or tug-the-nose really aim at defeating another person? Or could it be a demonstration of one's own endurance, showing that one can endure such an ordeal? Or is it a way of forming a relationship with the opponent, or an encounter of a grotesque nature with the opponent?

Our reflections on how to construct elementary body-anthropological categories on the basis of pull and tug raise critical questions about the naiveté of body cultural practises as well as about what we take for granted in everyday life. These questions require a deeper and more nuanced understanding of what human movement is, what fighting is, what human encounter in bodily action is, and, in this context, of what "sport" is.

It has been proposed that sport should be treated either in an aesthetic or in a moral connection (Møller 1999). This proposition can be seen in the context of a Kantian epistemology that fundamentally distinguishes, in a more nuanced way, however, between three different sets of questions regarding theoretical "pure knowledge", morality, and aesthetics. Immanuel Kant described these three kinds of transcendental ideas in his philosophical main works: "*Kritik der reinen Vernunft*" (1781), "*Kritik der praktischen Vernunft*" (1788) and "*Kritik der Urteilskraft*" (1790). On one level, human beings raise questions of "pure reason" about the truth: Is this true or false? On another level, there are questions of ethics: Is this good or bad? Questions about aesthetics follow a third logic: Is this beautiful or sublime, does it appeal to my delight or inspire feelings of revulsion (*Lust* or *Unlust*)? These three logics should not be confused with each other.

From this perspective, sport can be seen in different and contradictory ways, indeed. Sport can be viewed as a training ground for ethical behaviour, as the ideologists of educational gymnastics, such as Friedrich Ludwig Jahn, of public school sport, such as Thomas Arnold, and of Olympism, such as Pierre de Coubertin and Carl Diem, believed. No, argued others like Bert Brecht: sport is rather a matter of aesthetic perfection, which is fundamentally immune to moral judgments. Sport offers the sensuality of beauty and the sublime. From this perspective, the ethical arguments against doping are not convincing, as they transform an essentially aesthetic phenomenon into a moral problem (Møller 1999).

The dualistic argument that makes sport either an aesthetic or an ethical phenomenon fails to acknowledge the logic of "pure reason" as a third possibility: that sport can also be regarded as a culture of achievement, in accordance with the principle of measurement. What is accepted as success in sport is neither determined by aesthetic criteria – how beautiful the show is – nor by ethical criteria that determine to what degree sport presents a model of virtue. The criterion of a performance is what is measured in centimeters, grams or seconds, and the discourse about who has won and by what margin is a discourse of truth. Sport is a laboratory for producing faster, higher, stronger performances, or what Soviet theorists once called anthropomaximology. The results of sport may, but only secondarily, be evaluated as good or beautiful, but only the quantitative record is decisive. In this respect, sport is rather a ritual carried out in the spirit of Kant's notion of "pure reason".

The philosophical division between the true, the good and the beautiful can be used to analyse some current arguments about doping and sport by employing a method of contradiction. It does not, however, help to determine the "essence" of sport, because it does not tell us whether sport belongs to one of these categories or the other. Sport as a psychological and sociological phenomenon is characterised by varying combinations of the three elements that philosophy has defined. This is not only true for sport. Is mouth pull an aesthetic art or is it an ethical exercise? Is tug-of-war? The impossibility of formulating a convincing answer calls our attention to the fact that the Kantian categories were formulated in a pre-sociological and pre-psychological period of knowledge. This does not diminish Kant's intellectual importance. But it does relativise the use of his categories, once sociology and psychology begin to influence human self-reflection. Measured with "pure reason", ethical "practical

CHAPTER THREE

reason" and aesthetic "judgment", the phenomena of human life are complicated by sociological and psychological factors. Applying categories such as the true, the good and the beautiful on them in a direct way looks therefore somewhat simplistic or naive.

Is there help to be found in some sort of post-psychological, post-sociological philosophy? In fact, by invoking the epistemological contradiction between objectivity and subjectivity, we can define some existential dimensions of human movement culture. With a little help from Martin Buber (1923) we can ask what the objective "It" and what the subjective "I" in mouth pull are. In addition, we can raise questions about how meaningful the contradiction is between It and I, between objectivity and subjectivity, but also where the limitations of this binary construction are. Do they prompt us to think of a third concept, the relational "Thou" of play and games? In this way we can approach a deep psychology of movement.

It – The objective dimension of movement

Human movement can thus be seen as producing something. In modern sports, these products are performances and records. "Go for it!" Sport and modern gymnastics are predicated on such results. Indeed, this reification differentiates sport from older games and play. Tug-of-war is one illustration of this process.

Achievement and performance

When modern sport took on definitive modern forms at the end of the nineteenth century, its founders often regarded it as a "natural" prolongation of older popular practices involving games and competition. As these games traditionally included rope pulling, tug-of-war could also be regarded as sport, and as a sport with an especially long historical tradition. Its place in the new world of sports was, however, far from clear. Tug was sometimes treated as part of gymnastics (Georgens 1883, 155), but sometimes also connected with combat or fighting sports, as they were practised in military and police circles (Balck 1886/88, 516-517). In other cases, tug-of-war was regarded as a strength event (German *Kraftsport* or *Schwerathletik*), but was also put under the category of track-and-field (German *Leichtathletik*, Danish *fri idræt*) (Meyer 1908, 2, VI, 87).

Tug-of-war was, at any rate, an obvious candidate for the Olympic programme. From 1900 to 1920, there was rope-pulling at the Olympic Games, and at the 1900 Paris Games, a mixed Danish-Swedish team won the first gold medal in this event. After 1920, however, tug-of-war disappeared as an Olympic discipline and has never returned, despite the efforts of the Tug of War International Federation (Burat 1990; Wallechinsky 1992, 667-668; Crawford 1996).

This discontinuity shows that pull-and-tug competitions do not represent the modern performance principle. The game of pulling had to be transformed to adjust it to the sportive pattern of achievement. The sportive tug is no longer a trial of brute, "primitive" strength, but rather a systematic development of purpose-oriented skill and technique. Despite this transformation in the direction of sport, tug-of-war kept its distance from record-oriented sport. How is performance measured in a tug-of-war? The "record" for the longest tug event in history, as monitored by the Amateur Athletic Association and measured in 1938, was 8 minutes and 18,2 seconds. This was not so much a performance as a kind of curiosity. In tug-of-war, the fascination with "performance" is not focused on the quantified record.

From this perspective, the early difficulties involved in categorizing tug-of-war as a sport are illuminating. Whether tug is compared with ball-games and other gymnastic games such as *Turnspiel*, or with track-and-field events such as running, jumping and throwing, or with weightlifting and tossing the caber as an athletic event, or with a combat sport like wrestling, the objective, interpreted as performance, is different. Tug and pull do not correspond to the rationality of modern performance and achievement. It is not so easy to say what the "It" is, what this "sport" is supposed to produce.

It is likely that other features of tug-of-war have hindered the integration of this game into the Olympic canon, too. From popular culture, tug "sport" has inherited the grunting and grimacing of the actors, as well as the laughter. It approaches the grotesque in that the victors, at the moment of triumph, will probably fall on their arse. Strong men or women, snorting and groaning, and tumbling backwards on the grass, fit very well into a popular culture of play and carnival, connecting actors and spectators through the social convulsion of laughter. It does not, however, fit into the culture of achievement as it was developed by the industrial bourgeoisie, and it is still less suitable for Olympism and its strategy of assimilating sport to aristocratic norms and to a new type of "serious" elitist style. Doubts concerning the seriousness of tug sport may, in fact, have been amplified by an event at the Olympic Games in Paris 1900. After the official Olympic tug, a "friendly" tug was arranged for the American team which had not been allowed to participate. But the event broke up when American spectators rushed forward to join the game (Wallechinsky 1992, 667). Tug-of-war was, indeed, "something of a joke".

It is much more difficult to imagine mouth pull as an Olympic sport. A consistent application of technique and rational skill to the mouth pull would lead inevitably to mutual mutilation or self-mutilation. The idea of an "International Mouth Pull Federation" sounds strange, indeed. The "unserious" features of popular laughter and grotesque carnivalism stand

in the way of the "sportization" of this activity. And though the tugging –
or tearing-off – of the nose, ear or mouth may appear as "extreme", it
does not fall under the category of today's "extreme sport", either.

It is through their non-sportive features that mouth pull and tug-of-
war illustrate what sport is. Sport is not bodily movement and competition as such, but is rather a specific form of production, of producing
results, of a quantifiable outcome. It is an activity that is characterized by
growth and the maximizing of results. Sportive activity produces an
objective "It". Sport displays in its ritual forms the productivism of
industrial capitalist society.

Rules

Performance is not, however, the only form of reification that characterizes modern sport. Another form of its "It" is rules. "Do it this way" is the
message of ruled-ordered sport, a development that is typical of modern
gymnastics. Here what is of primary importance is not to produce a
result, but to complete a given movement "in the right way", the point of
sport being to enforce conformity with rules. Training is the regulation
and correction of movements. Ideally, the trainer or instructor, standing
face to face with the exercisers, possesses a panoptic overview and applies
the rules by commanding, inspecting and reviewing the gymnasts' movements.

While performance-oriented sport came to dominate in English, Scottish and North American sports, and became the international norm
during the twentieth century, early examples of rule-bound sport date
from the later eighteenth century in the form of Nordic gymnastics,
German gymnastics (*Turnen*) and Slavonic gymnastics (*Sokol*). These
were the forerunners of modern sport, later also opposing models to
competitive sport, and they remain an important undercurrent in today's
modern body culture. While performance-oriented sport reified results,
rule-ordered gymnastic sport reified movements by dissecting them into
their constituent parts. These movements were codified in choreo-
graphed patterns, which were further codified as gymnastic "systems".
Some of these systems were oriented more towards aesthetics, others
more towards physiological and anatomical rules. Modern social dance
developed similar patterns of steps and figures, parallel to those of military exercises, which had taken a geometrical form as early as in the sev-
enteenth century.

Rule-ordered sport was not simply antithetical to performance-oriented sport. The discipline of rules entered into performance-oriented
sport in the form of training and became another means for producing
the peak performance. Training in accordance with rules helped to create
a health-oriented sport as well as a sport that could serve educational

purposes. In sports pedagogy, for instance, the idea developed that the rule was central to the understanding of sport. Sport was in its educational essence a formation of character and training in accordance with rules. From this perspective, respecting the rules appears as the core value of sporting sociality, of learning through sport (Digel 1982).

Also Inuit games have come to the attention of educators as an example of rules for bodily training (Frey/Allen 1989). Rule-abiding Inuit games served the politics of identity in the Inuit societies, which were achieving cultural and political self-determination during the 1970 and 1980s. Among these games was mouth pull.

> *Equipment: None.*
> *Stance and Start: Both competitors stand side by side on set line. Inside feet are meeting. Each competitor grabs mouth of opponent with inside hand by going around the neck and grabbing outside corner of opponent's mouth with middle finger.*
>
> *Movement: On a signal, competitors try to pull opponent to their side of the line. Strongest mouth wins.*
>
> *Judging and Scoring: Wash hands before competition. Best out of three tries* (Keewatin 1989, 38).

These rules have a grotesque aspect. If they were strictly applied, they would produce mutilation. So the competitive pattern with its rules does not quite fit here. The rule of hygiene imposes further features of grotesque correctness. In fact, rules fail here because this tug does not require rules at all. The technique will best be transmitted mimetically, from face to face and from movement to movement. How it feels is enough regulation in itself. There is nothing like "correct implementation" in this game. And systematic training for mouth pull is meaningless, either as educational device or for the production of a peak performance.

This contrast becomes evident when we compare mouth pull with the sportifed tug-of-war. Transforming rope pulling into a sport required a remarkable set of codified rules, defining in detail weight classes, the size of the team, time limitations, the standardization of the field, restrictions on footwear, etc. The first rules of tug-of-war were drawn up in 1879 for the New York Athletic Club, and the AAA in England introduced its first rules in 1887. Conflicts arose at the 1908 Olympics in London, when, in the first round, the Liverpool Police pulled the US team over the line in a matter of seconds. The Americans protested that the Liverpudlians had used special illegal boots with steel cleats, spikes and heels, whilst the British replied that they were wearing standard police boots. The protest was disallowed and the Americans withdrew from the remainder of the competition (Wallechinsky 1992, 668).

Rules of a more technical kind were developed to rationalise the movements of tug-of-war. They regulated how the hands were to grasp the rope, the position of the body, time and rhythm of movement, the distribution of roles (anchorman) as well as strategy and tactics. Each of these rules increased the efficiency of the physical effort, and athletes were able to train for them separately. In this respect, the rules for gymnastic training were not an alternative to modern achievement sports, as the ideologists of gymnastics and advocates of sport have sometimes claimed (Guttmann 1994, 139-156). Rule-bound sport was the reverse side of sport as production. Both were subject to and united by reification.

Equipment and facilities

Performances and rules were the most important, but not the only, factors in the creation of modern body culture. Equipment and facilities also made innovation visible. Playthings and newly invented apparatuses were a starting point for the creation of modern children's play centred around toys. Similarly, the mechanization of sport led to a multiplication of apparatuses for existing activities. And to an increasing degree, newly invented devices also created new sports, from the "machine gymnastics" of the nineteenth century to roller skating, cycling and motor sport, and further to surfing, mountain biking, hang-gliding, inline skating, snow boarding and bungee jumping (Eichberg 1982, Vigarello 1988).

The games of pulling were never in a similar way dominated by technical equipment. For popular activities of pull and tug, people had earlier used simple implements such as the rope, the stick and the hand-grip, not more. And in modern times, devices of higher technological complexity did not take over to the same degree as they did in sport and gymnastics.

Facilities are another aspect of modern sportization. Whilst older games occupied certain areas of villages, landscapes or towns, periodically redefining the places of everyday life for festive occasions, the landscape of modern sports and physical education presented itself as a specialized space for permanent "functional" use. The "sportscape" consists of fields and halls for specific sportive monocultures. Highly specialized spaces for training exist side-by-side. The distinctions between different rules, between different systems of achievement, produced new and historically unique forms of spatial exclusivity (Bale 1994). This was part of an overall specialization within society at large, ranging from the school and the playground to the museum and the prison (Foucault 1975).

This colonizing of space would require a specialized space for the modern sport of tug-of-war or other forms of tugging and pulling. For example, a stage for mouth pulling could be erected before an amphitheatre for the spectators. Or the game could find its niche in the world of educational games, with the gymnastic hall hosting a pedagogical and enjoyable mouth pull. Or the event could be relegated to a museum, to be displayed there as a relic of "traditional Eskimo culture". Alternatively, and if we do not accept these segmentations, the mouth pull can be read as a living critique of sportive, pedagogical, and folkloristic space.

Function

On a more abstract level, there is "function". The "functional" roles of sport and games were invented in order to make them serve certain societal goals. Sports science ascribes to sport certain physiological functions related to health, a role in personal development and stress reduction, a role in promoting social integration and the reduction of violence, and a political role in preserving the actual state. The "functional" role of of dance is seen in terms of "socialization", "tension management", "adaptation to societal goals" and "integration." Architectural functionalism created the classical "functions" of residence, work, trade, leisure and traffic in order to justify strategies of urban segmentation.

Functionalism reached a new level in the sort of system theory espoused by Luhmann. System theory relates the administrative practice of sector division to some higher type of theoretical, "functional" logic, to economic, juridical, educational, political, religious, scientific, etc. functions that are said to be based on binary codes of global significance. In this model, sport serves originally medical and educational functions, which are determined by codes such as ill/healthy and educated/uneducated. But with the advent of modernity, sport has developed towards an autonomous functionality, following the sportive code of win-or-lose (Cachay 1988, Bette 1989), which, however, also has been declared as universal (Tangen 1997).

As accidental and artificial as these functions may look, the different approaches share a strategy of reification that is linked to a program of socio-political stabilization. The word "function" is derived from mathematical terminology and therefore has both "scientific" and "objective" connotations. Function is imagined as a quasi-thing or factor, an "It" of higher quality. The meaning of "function" oscillates somewhere between essence (*Wesen*), intention, purpose, aim, value, instrumental meaning, cause, reason, and driving force (*Triebkraft*). As is typical for a myth, the ambiguity of the notion is hidden away, so this term appears to be a convincing expression of objective truth. What the *Wesen* or essence of a thing is may be a mystery, but its "function" seems us to be clear. Function is, as Norbert Elias expressed it, a hidden notion of causality (*ein versteckter Ursachenbegriff*).

The reified "It" of the "function" is further characterized by a conservative undertone. Implicitly, the notion postulates some ideal, designates hegemonic societal goals as "functional," and rejects oppositional values as "dysfunctional". When existing relations of power are called "functional", they are withdrawn from conflict, naturalized and justified, whilst subversive dimensions are systematically neglected. "Function" is not what is installed by power, what can be disputed and changed on the base of alternative needs – function is function. It is true that the discourse of a "revolutionary function" is not unknown and has been tried now and then. But it cannot be accidental that functionalist reification predominantly goes hand in hand with endorsing the existing power structures.

What is the "function" of mouth pull? Does pull and tug contribute to health, personal development, stress reduction, social integration or tension management? The utilitarian functions of "training for work", "preparation for hunting" or "exercise for war" that the older ethnology/anthropology has ascribed to so-called "primitive" games are difficult to apply to mouth pull, as to many other games, including ball games. Here we may turn to the notion of the "fertility cult". This concept was developed by the earlier functionalism and has opened the door to some highly speculative ideas about "primitive" functionality. The finger in the smooth, moist and warm mouth of the partner may lead to psychoanalytical interpretations, as well ...

Functionalism is not only an academic luxury, it is a political term, as well. This is evident in the Western strategies of sport development aid for the developing world. The developmental theory of the functionalist mainstream recommends sport to non-Western countries as being instrumental to central "functions": the development of personality, social and political integration (nation building), identity formation, health, equality of opportunity and the satisfaction of basic needs (Digel 1989, 73-137). Native games have no place in this world of "functions", and it is with explicit reference to pulling games that developmental thinking denounces "folkloristic marginal activities"; they have – like *Fingerhakeln* (finger pull) – "hardly anything to do with sport and are therefore properly excluded from the reflection of the sport sciences" (Digel 1989, 165). While "function" may, indeed, help to exempt unwanted practices from critical reflection, it does not help us to understand movement culture.

Objectification, reification and the impossible game

The results of movement, the rules, the devices, the facilities and the functions – all have in common the fact that they give the impression of objectivity. The act of movement becomes an objective "It". What flows becomes a quasi-object. The mouth pull is instructive here because it shows how limited this perspective is. In this respect, mouth pull is not only harmless, but also (and paradoxically) subversive.

This critical perspective is not meant to suggest that objectification is an evil in and of itself. The relation between I and It is neither specifically

modern nor illegitimate as such. An objective movement such as the tri-
umphal gesture of a victorious athlete (which is not identical to modern
performance), the mimetic and repetitive transfer of bodily technique
(which is not the same as the rules of modern sport), the agreement to
meet and play at a particular time and place (which is not the same thing
as the modern facility) and the myth of what is good and bad (which is
not yet the modern "function") are much more deeply rooted in human
culture. The relation of the subject I to the objective world of the It is fundamental to being human. But this existential objectification took on a
new and expansive dynamic when modern performance and production
appeared, with their quantification of results, systems of rules, production of things and their standardization of the sportive space.

Industrial production gave new dimensions to the reification of life.
Reifying terms such as "function", "system", and "evolution" became a
mythical superstructure that came to dominate the discourse of modernity. "*Die Zwingherrschaft des wuchernden Es*" was established, "the dicta-
torship of the proliferating It", as Martin Buber (1923) called it. The
golem takes over – the robot servant makes itself the master of the human
being. Others called this *Entfremdung*, alienation.

Play and games offer living images of processes that otherwise are
described in highly abstract terms. One critical image is that of "the
impossible game", since many games are impossible to play if the players
really follow the rules. They are what we can call, with Jørn Møller, *den u-
lade-sig-gørlige leg* [the game that cannot be played]. If the rules for the
mouth pull were strictly applied – "the strongest mouth wins" – this
would lead to mutilation. Also games that involve running and catching,
as many forms of children's games, are impossible if they are performed
in a productivist way. If all of the participants are following the rules, running away as quickly as possible, the slowest runner will very soon lag
behind, perhaps in tears, and the game will come to an abrupt end. The
game lives off of continuation and flow. If the play process is to go on, this
can only happen against the rules, against the "fair" domination of speed.
Instead, the faster runner will approach the slower one, teasing her, pro-
voking him: "*Du kan ikke fange mig* – you can't catch me". It is in the
interest of the quicker runner to be caught. The game lives on the chance
the stronger runner gives to the weaker one. It is in the interest of all that
there be no loser. The rule is not the game. The flow of the game is in
contradiction to "performance." The game is what starts beyond the rules
and beyond the striving for performance – beyond the It.

I – The subjective dimension of movement

Beyond the It of objectification we find the subjectivity of the player, the
I. In movement, I experience something, I experience the other, I experi-

ence myself. Movement has a dimension that withdraws from objectification, from the It-relation.

Personal and situative experience

In pull, I experience *strength* as my strength: "I can". Force is felt as physical power, but also as a radiating energy, as my *inner force*. Mouth pull has a component of I-proof. I prove myself, my resistance and my perseverance. Can I stand it, can I endure it? In movement, the I enters into a relation to itself, to its Self. In the game, I enter into contact with my feelings.

The subjectivity of I-proof has been cultivated in different cultures in different ways. The Inuit practiced many exercises where, as in the case of mouth pull, the point was not so much to win over the other, but to endure. The difference between Inuit fist fighting and Western boxing is illustrative in this respect. In Inuit fighting, the opponent is not knocked down with a hard kick, but is slapped with the slack hand. This technique cannot produce a knock-out, but each fighter is challenged to endure: "You won't get me down – I can stand it". Inuit society traditionally cultivated the strong man, *nipitôrtoq*, whom nobody can force down. "Beat me!" he challenges all around. People are invited to box him, to tear his nose, to tousle his hair, but he remains stolid and just laughs.

This can be compared to the display of the strong man in Japanese sumo wrestling (Newton/Toff 1994) as well as the strong woman of *onna sumo* (Kaneda 1999). After a ritual preparation and a few seconds of action in the ring, the sumo fighters separate from each other with stolid faces. Their relaxed attitude proclaims: "I can", instead of the highly emotional Western drama that promotes "action against".

In the Western world, however, we experience a similar situation when the father challenges his small son: "Hit me!" The boy hits his father in the belly, the father laughs, and both have their pleasure. We are familiar with Bud Spencer's entertaining film version of the strong man confronted with all those who hit him in vain. The configuration of sport is different from this pattern. What the sportive fight cultivates as tension is in those hit-me games a demonstration of relaxation and of a strength, which takes the form of *laughter*.

Another experience involved in mouth pull concerns *intimacy*. The other is breaking through the limits of my body, as happens in different forms of wrestling, too. What is more, the other is sticking his hand into my mouth, at which point I may experience feelings of shame or disgust. Where is my integrity, where does my body end? The limits of my body are challenged from within. And within this bodily clash, *pain* arises. The grip of the other hurts me. I suffer and I resist. Still, in the interplay between pain and resistance, I feel *pleasure*, too. There is flow and energy. I laugh as I bring the action to a close.

The subjective experience of mouth pull is an experience of a *situation*. The event is here and now. I pull, I am pulled, pain and pleasure meet in the totality of the moment. The I has a situational presence similar to what happens in a dream and in love. The situation whose totality never can be caught in all of its dimensions presents an epistemological contrast to the structures and processes that can be objectified (Lefebvre 1959, 335-353, 637-655).

From Eigen-Sinn to epistemological solipsism

In the tension between It and I, modern epistemology has unfolded its main contradiction. Modern science of science consists typically of two major aspects: Analytical methods promise "objective" knowledge, the truth of It, while hermeneutical and phenomenological methods investigate the subjectivity of the I (Seiffert 1971). This apparent balance may, however, be deceiving. In the discourse of modernity, objectification is hegemonic, subjectivity at best tolerated.

Like modern reification, modern subjectification follows specific historical and societal dynamics. The modern state produces an individual who is subject to panoptical and disciplining strategies (Foucault 1975). The market produces the individual as a consumer who is going on his or her own way while choosing between offers. As individual, everyone is "the maker of one's own fortune": *I shop, therefore I am*. Identity appears as Self, and Self as identity, producing the illusion of sameness: I am I. I am myself.

Within the superstructure of mainstream discourses and interpretations, epistemological solipsism treats the human being as if she or he were alone in the world. The individual is the primary actor, and the social dimension is secondary. Sociologists say "individual and society" as if society somehow existed outside of the individual. (Norbert Elias built his figurational sociology against this separation – with very limited success, alas!) The sociology of "individualization" and "self-identity" translates this into the historical process of modernization and postulates that we are on the way to becoming our own *"Gesamtkunstwerk I"* (Beck 1998). The modern I that only refers to itself appears, as Martin Buber (1923) put it, as a ghost in the back of the modern It. Where the golem produces results, and nothing but results, the Ego flutters, a bodiless phantom of soul and mind, shadow-like through the factory of industrial capitalism.

The specific monumentalization of subjectivity and individuality in the process of modernity should, again, not obscure the fact, that the I is a basic relation of the human being. Like the I-It relation, the I-Self relation is existential. The person has a monological potential, the I has *Eigen-Sinn* – a meaning of its own. (In German, *Eigensinn* means both the singular importance of a human being, and a capricious, obstinate attitude).

It is a widespread stereotype that the pre-modern human being has no self or "I". This assumption conforms to the colonial myth that "the others" have "not yet" reached our level of subjective development. However, where people pull the mouth or tug the finger, the person is in practical relation to his or her self, the *eigensinnige* human being is being himself or herself by playing the game. Whether modern or pre-modern, whether Inuit or Danish, I experience strength and disgust, pain and pleasure, it is me who laughs and who is at the centre of "the moment". The I of personal experience is both human and universal. Modern subjectivity, by contrast, the pseudo-sovereignty of the individual, is historical. It is as historically specific as the individuality of choice in the supermarket.

Equality, inequality and in between

Paying attention to subjectivity in games helps us to gain a deeper understanding of human movement. It turns our attention to the difference between two sets of rules, which contradict each other under the aspect of equality. Pulling games illustrate this contrast. One model shows two equally strong parties pulling against each other in order to produce a fair outcome, to produce It. Rules aim at creating and guaranteeing the balance that makes the result fair. Though this pattern may look "natural" from a Western point of view, equality does not offer the only model of pulling. In another model, we see one person challenging the others, so that all pull against one. While there is a fundamental imbalance, this is not a mistake or cheating, it is the meaning of the game. The unequal hit-me game demonstrates the force of "myself".

But these two models do not tell the whole story. The contradiction is illuminating but incomplete. This is shown by games of the type known as *Brobrobrille*. *Brobrobrille* is one of the best known and most-practised children's games in Denmark. It combines song, catch and pull games. Two children form a bridge with their arms, and the other children walk or dance in a row under the bridge and around the two, singing:

> "*Bro bro brille, klokken ringer elleve.*
> *Kejseren står på sit høje, hvide slot,*
> *så sort som en kul, så hvidt som en kridt.*
> *Fare, fare krigsmand! Døden skal du lide.*
> *Den der kommer allersidst, skal i den sorte gryde.*
> *Første gang så la'r vi ham gå, anden gang gør vi ligeså.*
> *Tredje gang så ta'r vi ham og putter ham i gryden.*"

(Bridge bridge brille, the bell is ringing eleven.
The emperor stands on his high white castle,
as black as a coal, as white as chalk.
Go, go warrior, you shall suffer death.
He who comes last will go into the black kettle.
First time we let him go, second time just the same.
Third time we take him and put him into the kettle.)

One after the other, the children are caught by the two bridge persons and put "into the black kettle". They have to decide in secret between two alternative possibilities like "sun" and "moon", and take their place behind the respective bridge person who is, again secretly, named "moon" or "sun". In this way, two teams are formed which, finally, tug against each other. Embracing each other in a long line, the two rows pull their foremen "sun" and "moon" from each other as these hold each other's hands. The game ends when one team has tugged the other over a designated line. Similar games are known from other Scandinavian countries, from Belgium and the Netherlands. In Germany they play *"Das Brückenspiel"* and in England *"London Bridge"* (Tvermose 1931, 220-230).

As in the case of other types of joint pulling games, it is difficult to describe this activity exclusively in terms of the I-It or I-Self relationships. The result of the pull, the It, is not of central importance, the two teams being unequal in strength and randomly chosen. Nor does individual experience or proof of the I's strength play any apparent role, as it would in an endurance competition involving "the strong man". A third relationship appears here: togetherness, body-to-body contact, the interaction between I and You.

You – The relational dimension of movement

Games involve more than the production of an It and the subjectivity of the I. In games we actually meet each other. A game is an encounter: "Who are you – who am I?" In pull, we meet the other in multiple relationships: I meet the opponent on the other side of the rope, I meet the other on my own side, whom I embrace as in *Brobrobrille*; we meet the spectators, and – what is mostly overlooked – we meet the environment as otherness. This encounter should not be understood as simply idyllic. Encounter can also be disencounter, *Begegnung* can be *Vergegnung*, to put it into the idiom of Buber.

Encounter, the human being as With and Also

Pull – like other types of fight and combat – make us meet *nearness*: You are close to me. With your finger in my mouth, you break through the limits that define my intimate space. This proximity contrasts with the principle of distancing the other, which is characteristic of the politics of space in modern sport.

Your nearness may become sensible to me in my *pain*. Pain cannot be measured, that is why it is problematical for a medical system, which is programmed towards "It" and tries to overcome pain with drugs, doping or psychological tricks. On the other hand, pain is not only an individual feeling either, not only pure subjectivity of the monological "I". Pain comes into being by a collision between me and the world, in my collision with otherness. In this respect, pain is close to Buber's *Vergegnung*. You cannot prove your pain to me, but I can meet your pain in fellow-feeling. Mouth pull, fighting and combat also tell about this dialogical relationship.

We experience encounter and relation through rhythm. My movement is a rhythmical answer to your movement, and vice versa. In the to-and-fro of pull, the two opponents find a joint time together. In this respect, tug-of-war, like wrestling of the back-hold type, is a sort of dance. The rhythm fills the space between you and me.

The You-relation is manifest not only in the opposition of fighting, but also in the combination of forces, in togetherness through *body contact*. In Swedish games like "To pull the ox" and "To tame the mare", the players lie on the backs of their team-mates who crawl away from each other. And in the Breton game "*Ar vazh-a-benn*", each puller is held in the air by three or five comrades who help in the tugging (Møller 1990/91, 4, 20-22). This type of pull fight results in a collective result, which is amusing and sensual at the same time. "You" and "we" are linked together. I pull "with" the others and the result is "also" mine – the human being appears as With and Also, *Mitmensch* and *Auch-Mensch*.

In another way, encounter happens in the *show*, in the encounter of the players with their audience. Mouth pull and other tugging and fighting games are display, drama, expression and performance (Schechner 1993). The active player enters as an actor into dialogue with an audience. The game creates a scene, a situation of seeing and being seen. There is a reciprocal effect that occurs in the space between one's own grotesque body movement and the laughter of the others. Tug-of-war is said to be "famous for its vociferous participants and supporters" (James 2000, 401). In the show, there is interaction by means of collective crying and shouting. The noise expresses the high passions both on the field and amongst those watching – and in between.

On this basis, the Inuits have developed their drum dance into a kind of juridical theatre. Drum dance can be found in the Inuit culture both as festivity and as shamanic healing, but is also used as a technique for resolving conflict. A conflict arises, and instead of clashing in violence or calling for a decision by an authority, the two conflicting persons meet with the drum in hand and with well-prepared songs of insult, displaying their conflict to the public. By means of bodily and symbolic fighting, face-to-face with their audience of settler comrades, the Inuit were able to avoid the establishment of a formal power structure consisting of judge, chieftain, and state. The showing-up and showing-off of the dance contributed to the structural anarchy of the Inuit society. The spectator in this encounter is not passive, but contributes through his or her laughter and sympathy. The collective judge is an important partner in the game (Eichberg 1989).

Identity, non-identity, alterity

In the action of pulling and fighting, identity is expressed. Tugging displays the relation between We and You. The game is a bodily practice of nostrification: Who am I, who are you, who are *we*? This was expressed in the description of a Danish tug-of-war event in 1938:

> There were gigantic achievements. The blacksmiths quickly defeated the bakers, and the tailors could not long withstand the coal-heavers who weighed at least twice as much. But there arose a momentous competition between the dairy workers and the brewery men and – much to the distress of the agitators for abstinence – the beer won. The final was between the brewers and the coalmen, and here the brewery workers had "to bite the dust". "This is not at all surprising", said the captain of the coal-heavers. "You only carry the beer, but it is us who drink it" (Hansen 1993, 102).

The tug-of-war contest described in the Danish daily *Social Demokraten* was the highlight of *Fagenes Fest*, the workers' "festival of professions" in Copenhagen in 1938. This festival started in 1938 as an annual sporting event of the Danish workers' movement, stimulated by similar arrangements in France and Germany. It combined competitive sports events with more carnivalistic contests. Domestic servants ran matches with buckets and scrubbers, pottery workers engaged in matches with piles of plates on their heads, blacksmiths threw the hammer and socialist scouts ran obstacle races eating cream puffs on the way. As "we" and "you", the professional groups challenged each other, displaying themselves as identitary caricatures. Gender and age groups were also themes in the festivity. The demarcation by contrast – some of them assuming grotesque forms – were not intended, however, to incite one group against the other. The display of competing professions was ironic and self-affirmative at the same time, related to the image and identity of the worker, and that of the Danish worker. During the Second World War, when Nazi Germany occupied Denmark, *Fagenes Fest* could therefore develop into a demonstration of national togetherness, and it attracted at that time the largest spectatorship in its history (Hansen 1993).

The nostrification – the formation of *we*-ness – expressed in the tug was not only made complex by the overlapping of professional, gender-related, social class and national identities, but the game displayed non-identity at the same time. The "brewers" of the tug were both self and ironical non-self. They played a role. In a role game, movement is a sort of mask, just as one can play the king, the witch or the fool in carnival. Role is imitation of the other, whether a proud (re-) presentation, a caricatural mimesis, an impudent travesty – or a grimace of "the quite other". The grimace of mouth pull is not only a part of myself, but also an expression of otherness. I am another, this is what the distorted face tells about my own alterity. The Inuit culture is especially rich in elements of grimacing – grotesque, frightening and ridiculing, expressive and therapeutic. On this basis, modern Inuit theatre, like *Tukak* in Denmark, has developed a dramatic world of its own (Jørgensen 1979).

Festivity and environment, love and death

An important position between identity and non-identity is the play of gender, the *erotic* dimension of the game. The encounter in the You-game offers a broad spectre of erotic display. Games of flirting like *Brobrobrille* provide opportunities to touch and to be touched. Tugging and wrestling can display gender roles in caricatural forms up to and including the transvestite. The erotic is both an overlooked and effectively exploited aspect of sports (Guttmann 1996).

The great encounter of human life is *festivity*, the festive celebration when people say "you" to each other. Festivity puts rhythm into social time by lifting certain situations out of the flow of normality. At the same time it is by means of repetition that festivity creates ritual "holiness". By repeating the ritual encounter over and over again, the "I" faces the other as "You". In festivity, we get high in the here-and-now – together. In this respect, game and festivity are familial, maintaining a complex balance between unique situations and ritual repetition. And festivity is the social frame for play and games, from the mouth pull of Inuit winter festivity to the tug-of-war of the Danish workers' *Fagenes Fest*. The larger part of what modern sports historians have reconstructed as "sports history" is upon closer inspection nothing other than a history of festivity. It is true that the modern disciplinarity of sports made festivity tend to disappear but, as if through the back door, festivity reappears as the surrogate, as the show – the media event, the Olympic show.

In games, togetherness is also expressed in a more extensive, trans-human way: The human being has a relationship with the *environment*. Whether we tug the rope over the lawn of the suburb, or pull the finger in the smoky pub or as folklore for a touristic audience; whether Arctic people pull each other in the over-heated winter house, naked bodies close to each other, in a cloud of carbon dioxide, sweat and train-oil, surrounded by the deafening noise of the large skin-drums – by means of movement the human being meets something other which is larger than himself. Whether we build climbing architecture for children's games, shape thread-figures with the hand, roll the marble on the sandy ground or push the swing high up into the air; whether we run on the cinder track or swim in the lagoon, whether we explore "untouched" nature or challenge risky landscapes – by means of movement the human being says "you" to his and her environment. So games are a sort of living deep ecology.

Encounters and ecology may be misunderstood as idyllic, but this is not the whole story. In games like "To pull the cow to graze" (Danish *Græsse ko*), two opponents tug each other by a rope that they have tied around their necks. In some variations of the game, a pole or a fire is placed between them (Møller 1990/91, 4,19). You pull my head against the pole, I pull you into the flames ... if the game goes this far, the tug tells about *violence* and *death*. In some variants of Scandinavian wrestling, one could potentially break the back of the opponent. Whether it really goes that far is the suspenseful element of the game. Movement and games are also *dangerous*, wherein children can render themselves or others unconscious, creating fainting fits, while mature people climb dangerous rock faces or house facades, having drunk themselves senseless. Games can thus be risky endeavours (Sutton-Smith 1983, Le Breton 1991, Møller 1994).

This directs our attention to what sociology has called the contradiction between violence and civilization, even if this discussion has produced an often one-sided discourse. Traditionally, sociologists have opposed physical brutality to processes of self-discipline, pacification and civil non-violence. Violence is assigned here to an "early stage of civilization", the "phase of wildness" (Elias 1981). This violence was rediscovered in "the wild games of the Vikings" or constructed as such (Wahlqvist 1978). By contrast, civil pacification progressed in the course of modernization. On closer examination, however, pre-modern popular games may present a more nuanced picture than this one does. For compared, for example, with the level of violence in the early modern popular games of Sweden, modern sport appears to be somewhat more violent (Hellspong 2000).

Mouth pull raises questions about whether the dichotomy between violence and civilization is useful at all. Perhaps it says more about modern dualistic mythology. Beyond this dualism, games develop in an intermediary space. Violence and death are played out in the form of movement. By engaging in ritual interaction and repetition, human beings tell each other through their bodies that they are mortal – finite, but not alone in the world. It is precisely "the impossible game" that demonstrates this mortality. By means of the impossible game, people play out their finality. The human being is not only at home in the game, but also homeless – and a You, nevertheless.

How do people react to homelessness, pain and the proximity of death? People *laugh*. Laughter is also a way of saying "you". Its bodily expression is the convulsive interaction, a face-to-face reciprocity, from body to body. Laughter is catching, infectious, as though we were "possessed". Games are part of carnivalism, throwing into contrast the solemn productivity of "serious" Olympic sport. And on a very basic level, tickling tells the story of the more-than-individual body. I cannot tickle myself, but you can tickle me. For tickling, the I needs a You.

To touch and to be moved – dialogical relations

What games say through bodily display, language tries to express in its metaphorical way. Language lives on bodily movement, translating the living experiences of movement into the restricted code of words. The semantic dimension of words is, however, deeper than terms like semiotics, grammar, system and code, with their overrationalization (or underrationalization?), would have us believe. Whereas mouth pull and other tugging games are about touching, words respond through their diversity and etymological force (Goldschmidt 1988).

In mouth pull, as in other tug and wrestling games, we touch each other. "To touch" describes a bodily *tactile skill*, especially when it is carried out with the hand. Danish *at berøre, at røre ved, berøring*, correspond to German *berühren, Berührung*. *Touché* designates the act of making contact in fencing. The reflexive form, Danish *at røre sig*, German *sich rühren*, denotes at the same time the *movement* itself, "to move". In Swedish, *rörelse* is the bodily movement as such. In the non-reflexive form, Danish *at røre, at røre rundt* is a mostly *circular* movement, to stir – just like German *rühren, umrühren, herumrühren*. We *rører*, stir the dough for the cake, resulting in German *Rührkuchen*. To touch is also a *sensual feeling*. We speak of the sense of touch, along with the senses of seeing, hearing and smelling.

There is more in the game than physical movement and sensual experience. When we are touched, we are *emotionally* moved. Danish *at blive rørt, rørelse* means to be affected because something is touching – as in German *gerührt sein* and *Rührung* and French *être touché*. When we are touched, passion runs high, and we can be moved to tears. *Rührseligkeit*, sentimentality, is an intensified form of this emotion. From the sensual and emotional, it is not far to the eroticism of touch. And more: To touch denotes a social relation, a *contact*. Touch as *communication* has its bodily basis in what happens between wrestlers or pullers, but transfers this to a level of communicative interaction. In a literal sense, we promise to "stay in touch".

The bodily-emotional experience of touch can also be the basis of an *intellectual concern*: to touch on a topic. I can or cannot "touch on a certain question", by "touching something", I deal with it, and "everything he touches turns to gold". A combination of bodily, emotional and intellectual movement can be found where *der er røre* (Danish), where there is *excitation*, arousal or agitation. This may be spiritual movement, bodily turbulence or collective excitement.

Where this sort of movement is collectively organized, we approach what in Swedish is a *folkrörelse*, a *popular movement*. *Rörelse* – like Danish *bevægelse*, German *Bewegung* and French *mouvement* denotes by the same word a bodily as well as a social movement. *Rörelse* may be of religious, political or sportive character.

And finally, where there is touch and *berøring*, there is also *berøringsangst, fear of touch*. We may also be afraid of what happens in touching and movement, in being touched and being moved.

Towards an ex-centric theory of the body

Language thus attempts to contain the diversity of experience that is included in the movement of touch, in pull and tug. In any case, the game displays a relation. It is not by chance that in the German language *ziehen*, pull, and *Beziehung*, relation, have the same linguistic root. The "I" is not only able to conduct a monologue, but dialogue is existential, too.

The dialogical relation to "You" turns our attention to an alternative understanding of "the human", which has its centre not in the individual human being as individual, but in the intermediary space, the in-between. Where the I-perspective centralises, the You-perspective opens for the ex-centric dimension of "the human". The grimacing mouth pull and other eccentric tugs tell us about human ex-centricity – a social as well as a bodily story. The human being has no isolated existence. The human is not – not only, not primarily – inside the skin-body, but between human beings. And this is the case, not in a idealistic, bodiless sense, but in a concretely materialistic understanding. In tickling, "you" make me laugh, and you are necessary, because I cannot tickle myself. By playing hide-and-seek with the baby, *titte-bøh* in Danish, *Guck-guck* in German, we are "away" and feel the tension tickling in the belly, until the You reappears. By making noise – tam-tam – we create rhythm as a relation of resonance between you and me and the environment. Movement is a bodily medium showing, like the navel, breathing, and hearing, that the human being is not alone in the world (Sloterdijk 1998/99). The human being is an inter-body. Humanism is inter-humanism.

By means of the dialogical movement, we are able to transgress the dualism that has established itself in the theory of the body, confronting the "body we have" with the "body we are". This contrast, as it unfolded in German theory (Plessner 1941), can be illuminating and prolific, indeed. To have a body as opposed to being a body was based on a pre-existing dualism in the German language between the objective and material *Körper* and the subjective and spiritual *Leib*. *Körper* is It-body, *Leib* is I-body. American somatics has copied this by contrasting the objective "body" with the subjective "soma". But this is, again, not the whole story, as the Danish dualism of *krop/legeme* shows, which is constructed in another, more complex way (Eichberg 1995). It is only via the You that the body and movement of the human as fellow-human, *Mensch* as *Mitmensch*, can be described. Inter-body is the third.

From the inter-body and the dialogical situation "in-between" we can take the step back to the individual again. This becomes a new discovery: The I is not one. The I of the You-relation is someone other than the I of the It-relation (Buber 1923). The I of tickling – the I of I-You – is fundamentally different from the I that is achieving or following the rule, the I of I-It. And this is, again, someone other than the I of monological subjectivity and self-reference, of I-Self. If we compare the I of mouth pull and the I of sportive production, we follow what has been confirmed by centuries of Western thinking, but we remain far from the diversity of human existence and human sociality. The I of the human being is relative, relational and – at least – trialectical.

Two fundamentals of human life are in a special way illustrative of this relational existence: mortality and the existence of others. Death and *Mitmensch* show the limits of traditional Western humanism (Jespersen 2000) , and that is what games always have told about. The question is, where is sport to be found in this context? Is sport a story of human relational and dialogical life, too, in its modern edition, or is sport rather a counter-story about how to reify the other and to overcome death by prosthesis (Tibon-Cornillot 1979), by producing eternal forms of surrogate life and mortal engines (Hoberman 1992)?

So, what is sport, and where do we find ourselves when asking for its – non-existing – essence? I will try to sum this up in five theses.

1. Sport is neither universal nor does it have an essence. Sport is *culturally* specific and *relative*.
2. The analysis of this cultural relativity of sports leads towards a body anthropology describing *sociality inside the body*. Sociality is not only somewhere above, but inside of bodily practice. We thereby get in touch with a deep psychology, describing society inside the movement of the soul and of the feelings, as well.
3. There is nothing elementary or simple in movement, neither in run-

ning, jumping or throwing nor in pull or tug. The body is not simple, but a field of tension between the objective, the subjective and the *dialogical*. As a living body, the body is relative also in this respect.

4. If we understand the body as the material base of human existence, humanism is revealed as *inter-humanism*. The historian, sociologist or psychologist of sport, by working on the *ex-centric* dimension of bodily practice, delivers a picture of the grotesque, eccentric side of human existence.

5. This is not just a philosophical game, but a *political* one, as well. The modern production of performances is an invitation to totalitarian anthropomaximology, producing a freak circus plus pedagogy, mortal engines and the prosthesis-body of the future. This is a political choice. And games are not only forerunners or accompaniments, marginal relics or ersatz forms of sport, but also alternatives. There is *contradiction* in the field of body movement and sport.

Pulling the Christmas tree

The perspective provided by contradiction, ex-centricity and dialogical action helps us to approach concrete games, whether they are known around the world and standardized, as in sport, or marginal and local. One of the latter is the game of Pulling the Christmas Tree. It was practiced in a village school in Zealand, Denmark around 1950, as recalled by Jørn Møller, who was a schoolboy at that time and is today a leading scholar of play and games. On a certain day between Christmas and New Year, pupils and teachers would meet in their school to participate in a festivity, after which the Christmas tree would be removed. This was the task of the custodian. The children, however, did not like to see the tree disappear. On one occasion it happened that they took hold of the tree in order to prevent the caretaker from doing his job. They wanted the festivity to continue, and this developed into a pulling contest, a sort of tug-of-war. Parents who were present at the event entered into the action: Didn't the festivity have to come to an end sooner or later, and didn't order and cleanness have to be restored?! That is why some grown-ups pulled alongside the custodian, whilst others engaged on the side of their children. The result of this episode was a game of pull that became an annual event.

In Pulling the Christmas Tree, different elements of popular culture met and intertwined. The pulling competition was the bodily activity from which other dimensions grew. Certain roles – of pupils, custodian, teachers and parents – constituted the social relations. And a living story took form, telling about festivity and the tree, about tradition and innovation, about conflict, opposition and cooperative action. In short, the game was revealed to be nothing less than a poetic history of life itself.

Through the medium of bodily action, this event tells about accepting and cultivating difference, about life with contradiction and togetherness, about conflict and belonging.

References

Arlott, John 1975 (ed.). *The Oxford Companion to Sports & Games*. London: Oxford University Press.

Balck, Viktor ed. (1886/88). *Illustrerad Idrottsbok*. Vol.1-3, Stockholm: C.E.Fritze.

Bale, John (1994). *Landscapes of Modern Sports*. Leicester: Leicester University Press.

Beck, Ulrich (1998). "Gesamtkunstwerk Ich." In: Richard van Dülmen (ed.): *Erfindung des Menschen*. Wien: Böhlau. Pp.637-654.

Bette, Karl-Heinrich (1989). *Körperspuren. Zur Semantik und Paradoxie moderner Körperlichkeit*. Berlin: de Gruyter.

Buber, Martin (1923). *Ich und Du*. – In English: *I and Thou*. New York: Collier 1986 (first 1937).

Burat, Tavo (1990). "Il tiro alla fune." In: *Lo joà e les omo*, Aosta/Italy, 7, 37-46.

Cachay, Klaus (1988). *Sport und Gesellschaft. Zur Ausdifferenzierung einer Funktion und ihrer Folgen*. Schorndorf: Hofmann.

Crawford, Scott A.G.M. (1996). "Tug of war." In: David Levinson/Karen Christensen (eds.): *Encyclopedia of World Sport*. Santa Barbara: ABC-CLIO. Pp.1107-1110.

Digel, Helmut (1982). *Sport verstehen und gestalten*. Reinbek: Rowohlt.

Digel, Helmut/Peter Fornoff (1989). *Sport in der Entwicklungszusammenarbeit*. (= Forschungsberichte des Bundesministeriums für wirtschaftliche Zusammenarbeit. 96) Köln: Weltforum.

Dufaitre, Anne (1989) Traditional games. Preliminary observations on the preparation of a national or regional catalogue or inventory. (= Memorandum ACDDS 26.89) Strasbourg: Council of Europe.

Eichberg, Henning (1982). "Stopwatch, horizontal bar, gymnasium: The technologizing of sports in the 18th and early 19th centuries." In: *Journal of the Philosophy of Sport* 9, pp.43-59.

Eichberg, Henning (1983). "Einheit oder Vielfalt am Ball? Zur Kulturgeschichte des Spiels am Beispiel der Inuit und der Altisländer." In: Ommo Grupe et al. (eds.): *Spiel – Spiele – Spielen*. Schorndorf: Hofmann. Pp.131-153.

Eichberg, Henning (1990). "Stronger, funnier, deadlier: Track and field on the way to the ritual of the record." In: John Marshall Carter/Arnd Krüger (eds.): *Ritual and Record. Sports Records and Quantification in Pre-Modern Societies*. New York: Greenwood 1990. Pp. 123-34.

Eichberg, Henning (1989). "Trommeltanz der Inuit – Lachkultur und kollektive Vibration." In: Eichberg/Jørn Hansen (eds.): *Körperkulturen und Identität*. Münster: Lit. Pp.51-64.

Eichberg, Henning (1995). "Body, Soma – and Nothing Else? Bodies in Language." In: *Sport Science Review*, Champaign/Ill., 4:1, pp.5-25.

Eichberg, Henning (1997). "Otherness in Encounter. Thinking Folk Identity, Democracy and Civil Society with the Help of Martin Buber." In: Ove Korsgaard (ed.): *Adult Learning and the Challenge of the 21st Century*. Odense: Odense Universitetsforlag, pp.88-99.

Elias, Norbert (1981). "Zivilisation und Gewalt." In: *Ästhetik und Kommunikation*, Berlin, 10:43, pp.5-12.

Endrei, Walter/László Zolnay (1986). *Fun and Games in Old Europe*. Budapest: Corvina.

Floc'h, Marcel/Fanch Peru (1987). *C'hoariou Breizh. Jeux traditionnels de Bretagne.* Rennes: Institut Culturel de Bretagne.

Foucault, Michel (1975). *Surveiller et punir.* Paris. – In English: *Discipline and Punish.* Harmondsworth: Penguin.

Frey, Richard D./Mike Allen (1989). "Alaskan native games – A cross-cultural addition to the physical education curriculum." In: *Journal of Physical Education, Recreation and Dance,* Nov./Dec., pp.21-24.

Georgens, Jan Daniel (1883) (ed.): *Illustrirtes Sport-Buch.* Leipzig, Berlin: Otto Spamer. New ed. Münster: Lit, no year (1980s).

Goldschmidt, Georges-Arthur (1988). *Quand Freud voit la mer – Freud et la langue allemande.* Paris: Buchet/Chastel. – In German: *Als Freud das Meer sah. Freud und die deutsche Sprache.* Zürich: Ammann 1999.

Grunfeld, Frederic V. et al. (1975). *Spelletjes uit de hele Wereld.* Amstelveen: Plenary Publications.

Gutsmuths (1793). *Gymnastik für die Jugend.* Schnepfenthal. Reprint (= Quellenbücher der Leibesübungen. 1) Dresden: Limpert 1928.

Guttmann, Allen (1994). *Games and Empires. Modern Sports and Cultural Imperialism.* New York: Columbia University Press.

Guttmann, Allen (1996). *The Erotic in Sports.* New York: Columbia University Press.

Hansen, Jørn (1993). "Fagenes Fest. Working class culture and sport." In: Knut Dietrich/Henning Eichberg (eds.): *Körpersprache. Über Identität und Konflikt.* Frankfurt/Main: Afra. Pp.97-129.

Hellspong, Mats (2000a). *Den folkliga idrotten. Studier i det svenska bondesamhällets idrotter och fysiska lekar under 1700- och 1800-tallet.* Stockholm: Nordiska Museets Forlag.

Hellspong, Mats (2000b). "Våldets plats i den traditionella svenska idrotten." In: Johan R. Norberg (ed.): *Studier i idrott, historia och samhälle.* Festschrift for Jan Lindroth. Stockholm: HLS. Pp.63-73.

Hoberman, John (1992) *Mortal Engines. The Science of Performance and the Dehumanization of Sport.* New York: The Free Press.

Howell, Reet (1986). "Traditional sports, Oceania." In: David Levinson/Karen Christensen (eds.): *Encyclopedia of World Sport.* Santa Barbara: ABC-CLIO. Pp.1083-1093.

Hvormed skal jeg more mig? Samling af Lege og Beskjeftigelser for Børn og unge Mennesker, som kunne tjene til at uddanne Legemet eller skærpe Forstanden. Copenhagen: Pio 1861. (After the English: *The Boy's Own Book.*)

Idrætten i Grønland. Festschrift for the 25th anniversary of Grønlands Idræts-Forbund. No place (Greenland) 1978.

James, Trevor (2000). "Tug of war." In: Richard Cox/Grant Jarvie/Wray Vamplew (eds.): *Encyclopedia of British Sport.* Oxford: ABC-CLIO. Pp.401-402.

Jarvie, Grant (1991). *Highland Games. The Making of the Myth.* Edinburgh: Edinburgh University Press.

Jensen, Bent (1965). *Eskimoisk festlighed.* Copenhagen.

Jespersen, Ejgil (2000). "Døden og medmennesket i spejldans – mellem ånd og frihed." In: *Kompetence og demokrati.* Vingsted: DGI. Pp.15-22.

Jørgensen, Ole (1979). *Tukak'teatret – Eskimoisk trommesang.* DK: Tukak.

Kaneda, Eiko (1999). "Trends in Traditional Women's Sumo in Japan." In: *International Journal of the History of Sport,* 16:3, pp.113-119.

Keewatin Inuit Associations: *Inuit Games.* Originally published by the Department of Education, Regional Ressource Center, Government of N.W.T. Rankin Inlet 1989.

Korsgaard, Ove (1986). *Kredsgang. Grundtvig som bokser.* Copenhagen: Gyldendal.

Larsen, Helge (1972). "Sport hos eskimoerne." In: HENNING NIELSEN (ed.): *For sportens skyld.* Copenhagen, pp.117-127.

Le Breton, David (1991). *Passions du risque.* Paris: Métaillé.

LeFebvre, Henri 1959: *La somme et le reste.* Paris: La Neuf de Paris, vols.1-2.

Mauss, Marcel/Henri Beuchat (1904/05). "Essai sur les variations saisonnières des sociétés Eskimos." In: *L'année sociologique,* 9, 39-132. – In English: *Seasonal Variations of the Eskimo. A Study in Social Morphology.* London: Henley 1979.

Meyer, A.C. (ed.) (1908). *Idrætsbogen.* Vol.1-2, Copenhagen: Chr. Erichsen.

Møller, Jørn (1984). "Sports and Old Village Games in Denmark." In: *Canadian Journal of History of Sport,* 15:2, pp.19-29.

Møller, Jørn 1990/91: *Gamle idrætslege i Danmark.* New ed. Gerlev: Idrætshistorisk Værksted 1997, Vols.1-4.

Møller, Jørn (1996). "Klavremaskiner og trækfugle i det kasteløse Danmark." In: *Idrætshistorisk Årbog,* 12, 9-18.

Møller, Verner et al. (eds.) (1994). *Hooked. Om vanvid og æstetik i sport og kropskultur.* Odense: Odense Universitetsforlag.

Møller, Verner (1999). *Dopingdjævlen – analyse af en hed debat.* Copenhagen: Gyldendal.

Newton, Clyde/Gerald J. Toff (1994). *Dynamic Sumo.* Tokyo: Kodansha International.

Novak, Helmut (1989). *Schottische "Highland Games". Traditioneller Volkssport einer ethnischen Minderheit im Wandel der Zeit.* (= Düsseldorfer sportwissenschaftliche Studien. 4) Düsseldorf: Institut für Sportwissenschaft der Universität.

Plessner, Helmuth (1941). "Lachen und Weinen." Bern. In: Plessner: *Gesammelte Schriften.* Vol.7, Frankfurt/Main: Suhrkamp 1982. Pp.201-387.

Schechner, Richard (1993). *The Future of Ritual. Writings on Culture and Performance.* London, New York: Routledge.

Seiffert, Helmut (1971). *Einführung in die Wissenschaftstheorie.* München: Beck, vols.1-2.

Sloterdijk, Peter (1998-99). *Sphären.* Bd.1-2. Frankfurt/Main: Suhrkamp.

Stejskal, Maximilian (1954). *Folklig idrott.* Helsingfors. Doctor dissertation at the University of Åbo.

Sutton-Smith, Brian (1983). "Die Idealisierung des Spiels." In: OMMO GRUPE u.a. (eds.): *Spiel – Spiele – Spielen.* Schorndorf: Hofmann. Pp.60-75.

Tangen, Jan Ove (1997). *Samfunnets idrett. En sosiologisk analyse av idrett som sosialt system, dets evolusjon og funksjon fra arkaisk til moderne tid.* Bø: District University of Telemark. Phil. doctor dissertation at the University of Oslo.

Thisted, Kirsten (1997). *Jens Kreutzmann. Fortællinger og akvareller.* Nuuk: Atuakkiorfik.

Tibon-Cornillot, Michel (1979). "Von der Schminke zu den Prothesen. Elemente einer Theorie zwischen dem Aussen und dem Innen des Körpers." In: *Tumult,* no.2, pp.25-46.

Tvermose Thyregod, S. (1931). *Danmarks Sanglege.* Copenhagen: Schønberg.

Ulf, Christoph (1981). "Sport bei den Naturvölkern." In: Ingomar Weiler: *Der Sport bei den Völkern der alten Welt.* Darmstadt: Wissenschaftliche Buchgesellschaft. Pp.14-52.

Vigarello, Georges (1988). *Une histoire culturelle du sport. Techniques d'hier ... et d'aujourd'hui.* Paris: Robert Laffon.

Wahlqvist, Bertil (1979). *Vikingarnas vilda lekar.* Stockholm 1978. – In Danish: *Barsk idræt. Sport i vikingetiden.* DK: Hamlet.

Wallechinsky, David (1992). *The Complete Book of the Olympics.* London: Aurum.

Some Tug-of-War Websites:
British Tug-of-War Association: www.tugofwar.co.uk
Germany: www.tauziehen.de
Scotland: www.scottishtugofwar.co.uk

Acknowledgement:
Thanks to Jørn Møller for useful hints.

A Geographical Theory of Sport

John Bale

> The craze for the word 'space' ... expresses ... not only the themes that haunt the contemporary era ... but also the abstraction that corrodes and threatens them (Augé 1995).

Introduction

Geographical writing on sport has grown substantially in recent years. Such studies have spanned a variety of approaches but to date little has been done to present a geographical theory of sport. This lack of theorisation contrasts, for example, with work in sociology, philosophy and psychology where interpretations of sport have been rooted in several theoretical foundations. The purpose of the present essay is to speculate (as an essay should) about a geographic theory of sport that focuses on two themes central to sport, those of "fair play" and "achievement". Additionally I draw on geometry and science as two additional essences of modern achievement sport. I focus on the geographical scale of the field of "play" or the stadium – the site (rather than the location) of sport. My work is inspired by Edward Relph's (1976) notion of "placelessness", Henri Lebebvre's (1991) notion of "abstract space" and as Marc Augé (1995) puts it, "non-place." In theory, I suggest, the essence of the sport place is that it is "placeless" – a pure space. It is to this that I now turn.

Toward a geographical theory of sport

Discussions about the rationale or basis for a geographical theory of sport are few and far between. It is worth noting, however, that in drawing attention to the distinction between sport and recreation or leisure, the cultural geographer Philip Wagner argued that there was nothing natural about sports (by which he meant "achievement sports") and that as a result they are acted out in "an entire class of very closely defined conventionalised places" (Wagner 1981). Wagner's little-read paper is important because it basically defined sport (as opposed to recreation or leisure) *from an essentially geographic perspective*. The locations and landscapes of sportised body cultures are basically the outcome of its achievement orientation. Achievement orientation is not central to play or recreation and the landscapes and locations of these activities are therefore different. In modern sport measures of achievement are quantified, ranked, tabulated, averaged and recorded. This is most evident in sports like track and field, swimming and cycling in which science and technology have progressively refined the ability to record performances to at least a thousandth of a second. Beyond time-keeping, measurement is central to the definition of the space in which sport takes place.

My model – which might be a better way to present it – has one basic theorem – *that the sport landscape ought to be one of placelessness*. Note that this is a model of what 'ought to be'; it is a normative model that, in this case, is founded on the norms of sport itself. These norms provide the logic behind the model. With normative models it would be tilting at windmills to explore whether they fit the real world since the model is based on "what ought to be" rather than "what is". On the other hand, it is possible that the real world (in this case the "landscape" of sport) may be getting closer to the model, indicating that the model has some predictive qualities. If the world does not fit the model, it does not infer that the model is wrong; rather, it is the world that needs correcting in order to meet the norms of the model, assuming that the norms are widely subscribed to. In exploring the landscape of sport, I predict that the norms of sport logically encourage a "placeless", sanitised and sterile landscape (an appropriate metaphor would be the laboratory) and I conclude that over time there has been a tendency for sport places to become increasingly placeless. At the same time, however, I note that there has been a counter-tendency to retain a degree of place*ful*ness. There is, therefore, a tension between place and placelessness.

Placelessness can be summarised as the existence of homogeneous and standardised landscapes that diminish the local specificity and variety of places that characterised pre-industrial societies. It is reflected in what is often felt to be a growing 'sameness' in society (Relph 1976). As Lefebvre (1991) observes, 'abstract space [is] formal and quantitative, it erases distinctions'. In most areas of life where placelessness exists it seems to result from factors *extrinsic* to the activity upon which it is imposed. For example, McDonald's restaurants do not *have* to be the same in order for hamburgers to be produced. Likewise, suburban houses do not *have* to be the same for purposes of residential occupation. High rise buildings do not *have* to be standardised for office work to take place. It may be more efficient and more rational but it is not absolutely necessary. Placelessness in such contexts exists primarily for commercial, planning or design reasons. It is not intrinsic to the activities carried out at the places. In sports and in the production of sports spaces, on the other hand, I will argue that placelessness *is* intrinsic to the activity involved. It is part of the norms of sport, a part – often hidden – in its underlying (and sometimes conflicting) ideologies of fair play and achievement orientation.

My basic thesis is that the logic of achievement sport seeks to eliminate place (a unique area or peopled space) and replace it with space – or 'non-place' or placelessness. In sport the pressures are not to produce regional inflexions in the landscape (except in a superficial sense) but instead to move steadily towards the elimination of place-to-place differences. Such an assertion is based on the two concepts central to professional sport; these are *fair play* and *achievement orientation*. Each of these can be examined in turn.

Fair Play

The notion of fair play was established in sport in the 1850s. "Fair play" included the establishment of common rules, mainly referring to behaviour but also to the space on which sport was played. The most basic spatial rule was the imposition of a boundary that marked the field of play and explicitly served to signify a line of segregation between players and spectators. Inside the line, the space was "purified", being purged of spectators so that they could no longer wander on to an ill-defined playing space and interfere with the players and the progress of the game. It was a form of territorialisation, of power over people and space (Sack 1986). This was a way of making sport a fairer game. No such rules, however, were made in relation to place. There could be grandstands or open fields; spectators could number anything from 100,000 or more to 10 or less. Hence, in sport we have rules that clearly specify the spatial dimensions of the "play" later, "work") area but the details of the surrounding landscape ensemble – including the spectators – were left unspecified. If the *spaces* of sport were different from game to game, the outcome might be more laughable and this did, of course, exist in pre-modern, less serious sport-like forms. In a sense, playing with the body in pre-sportised body cultures were practices that were more akin to art than science; they were unplanned and unscripted, recorded orally and not standardised. Although they were games there was no 'game-plan'. A non-specialised sport landscape was occupied by non-specialised bodies, the presence of the grotesque body was found in the less serious landscapes in which such activities were practised. With the growing seriousness of the game came the growing seriousness of the landscape in which it took place.

Modern achievement sport is a world of geometry. For most sports the spatial parameters are very precisely defined. In the case of some sports (for example, football) the prescribed spatial extent of the pitch does vary slightly but the geometry and size of segments on the field of play are precisely defined and standardised. Given the limited margins within which the size of the pitch is allowed to vary, team managers have, nevertheless, been known to alter the width and/or length for games against particular opponents. The "space" of the Wembley pitch was often said to disadvantage certain teams. This seems to contravene the logic of fair play. For the ethos of fair play to be satisfied each space (and, I suggest later, each place) upon which a given sport occurs should logically be the same; otherwise, one participant or team would be unfairly advantaged.

An example of such an unfair advantage – though not often thought of as crossing the boundary of fair play – lies in the case of downhill skiers who live in, say Austria, and compete with those who live in, say, Denmark. Obviously, the former are widely thought to have an unfair advantage, but it is one that is tolerated by those who run the sport and many would argue that it is not necessarily unfair. As Roger Gardner (1995) argues, however, this claim 'would at least seem to suggest more analysis: because, at this point in time, such advantages do not seem to be *clearly* fair either'. An analogous example from football would be one in which the topographic nature of fields of play differed. Hence, a club with a pitch possessing an idiosyncratic slope, for example, is often deemed to possess and 'unfair advantage' over its opponents during the playing of home games. Let me take this argument a little further with another hypothetical example from football. Assume that a national football federation allowed clubs to play on either natural or synthetic surfaces. Assume also that only two clubs retained natural (grass) surfaces. Would it be "fair play" when these two clubs played every other club in the league? There seems to be a strong case to say that it would not and that the sport authorities should logically prescribe the same surface for all clubs. For fair play to be achieved, therefore, I am initially suggesting that the surface of the playing field should be – literally – even. This view has been explicated forcefully by the philosopher Paul Weiss. Though couched in the context of track and field athletics its general idea applies also to sport per se:

> ideally a normal set of conditions for a race is one in which there are no turns, no wind, no interference, no interval between signal and start, and no irregularities to the track – in short no deviations from a standard situation' (Weiss, 1986).

Replace the word "race" by "game" and it seems logical that such a "standard situation" should also apply in any sport. Weiss's "standard situations" are almost synonymous with the word "placelessness".

Achievement

A crucial characteristic of modern sport which distinguishes it from both its folk-game antecedents and recreation is its achievement orientation and its associated seeking after records, quantified and produced scientifically. For records and "progress" to be meaningful, each space where a performance may be achieved should be the same – exactly the same – or measurement of such progress would be impossible. The "production" of a record *requires* placelessness.

Here is the sporting analogue of the isotropic plane, the homogeneous surface, of the theoretical geographer Walter Christaller (or the "machine for sport" *pace* Le Corbusier). The plane is more than a metaphor as the character of the Astroturf football field, the scientifically regulated surface of an ice rink, or a synthetic running track will attest. The plane surface provides the rational solution to the problems of variety and individuality imposed by place. Indeed, although (as noted above) the size of soccer pitches vary, the spatial dimensions of points and segments on sport pitches are precisely prescribed; penalty area, centre circles, the penalty sport and the half way line have all quite precisely quantified dimensions. For the game to make sense, they must be the same on every football field in the world. Given these spatial regularities, progress in the tactical development of the game can take place. Skills can be developed which would be much more difficult if the spatial configurations of sport fields differed from place to place. In such ways geometry triumphs over space, segmenting it and territorializing it.

Science not only serves to segment sports space. It is also seen to triumph over nature and considerable pressure exists to eliminate nature from the sports landscape. Environmental interference in a sport match can be unfair. A strong wind blowing only during the second half of a match puts one of the teams at a disadvantage. This, and other kinds of environmental interference can be eliminated by moving sport indoors, a common tendency at the present time in North America and elsewhere. The introduction of prescribed artificial surfaces may lead to further predictability and placelessness. Until then, the sophisticated bio-chemistry of "turf science" seeks to provide surfaces which, in effect, differ from each other as little as possible and, at the same time, encourage progress in technical skills.

So far I have suggested that there is a tendency to eliminate certain environmental factors in order to subscribe to the logic of "fair play" and the protocols of achievement sport. I believe that there is considerable evidence that the sport landscape – at least, the field of "play" – is becoming more predictable, and hence more placeless. Contributors to football fanzines bemoan the "container architecture" of their stadiums and the sameness of the sport environment and philosophers of sport arrive at a similar prediction for the logical landscape of achievement sport. However, the place-making qualities of sport's milieu are difficult to deny – and to resist. Although football spectators may have been prevented from encroaching on the field of play with the inscribing of the white line around it in 1882, they still, literally, present "noise" with respect to my proposed theory. It is to the fans, therefore, that I now turn.

The "problem" of spectators

It is now appropriate to return more explicitly to the role of fandom in all this. In the English edition of Marc Augé's *Non-Places*, it is noted that "a space which cannot be defined as relational, or historical, or concerned with identity will be a non-place" (Augé, 1995). According to the norms of sport, sport spaces should not be concerned with identity because identification with them would create advantages for the home team. Yet sport is widely regarded as fostering identity, local and national. Sport is "representational".

Spectators at sports events create a problem for my theory of sport as a model of placelessness because, as noted above, in even the most sterile stadium the crowd acts as a form of "noise", creating a place out of nothing. The modern partisan spectator, in many sports, also creates problems for the notion of "fair play". Crowds at team sports undeniably influence performance; they contribute greatly to the "home-field advantage", even in the domed stadium; their Bakhtin-like carnivalism (as Richard Giulianotti has theorised the behaviour of Scottish – though not English – football fans) may contribute more to topophilia (a love of place – see Tuan 1974) than to placelessness (Giulianotti, 1991). It is the crowd that produces a "home field advantage" in the most sterile of environments – in sports like ice hockey and basketball. (Schwartz & Barsky, 1977; Zeller & Jurkovac, 1989). The enhanced home field advantage in such situations has been attributed to the closeness and involvement of the crowd.

In the early days of modern sports the fixed boundaries which now exist between spectators and players were absent. The explicit white line separating players from spectators was not introduced in soccer until a few years after the playing area had been designation by the four points, signifying the corners of the field of play (Bale 1995). Hence, although the spatial parameters were established in 1863, the insistence on a marked line did not occur until 1882. The boundary *communicates* the notion of territoriality – the imposition of power over space by point and lines, segments and arcs (Sack, 1986). Territoriality may therefore be seen as a way of solving the problem of spectator interference in sports. The boundary line did not prevent aural interference with play, however, which would logically help to favour the home team. For this reason early applause was directed at the visiting team in order to accord with the ethics of fair play. This "gentlemanly" conduct gradually disappeared with partisanship in the place-focus of many team games. What could have become sports *spaces* were clearly reclaimed as meaningful *places* by the crowd. The sports arena was not a space where one discriminatingly attended a "performance"; it became a meaningful place to support "our" team.

Such crowd interference reveals the liminality of sports space (Shore

1995). In many sports the spatial boundaries are constantly (and in some cases, deliberately) being violated. The crowd involvement, which makes the nature of boundaries in sports such a good example of liminal space – neither one thing or the other or a world betwixt and between playing and spectating – is not present in all sports, nor has it always been present in sports where it is currently found. We may have a synthetic isotropic plane, we have a territorialised space, but because of the place-making quality of people as sports spectators it might seem that my emphasis on placelessness has been misplaced. What seems to exist instead is a constant tension between place and space in an activity where placelessness would seem to be logically paramount. However, my story does not end here and while placelessness might typify modernity it is the sportsworld of the post-modern, as reflected in the writing of Jean Baudrillard and Paul Virilio, that I now turn.

In *The Transparency of Evil* Baudrillard (1993) refers to the Heysel disaster of 1989 and other negative aspects of sport stadiums. At Heysel sport was perverted into violence. In Baudrillard's words, "there is always the danger that this kind of transition may occur, that spectators may cease to be spectators and slip into the role of victims or murderers, that sport may cease to be sport and be transformed into terrorism: that is why the public must simply be eliminated, to ensure that the only event occurring is strictly *televisual* in nature" (Baudrillard, 1993). In Baudrillardian sport, however, the expulsion of spectators from stadiums also serves to 'ensure the *objective conduct of the match*, ... in ... a transparent form of public space from which all the actors have been withdrawn' (Baudrillard, 1993, emphasis added). The withdrawal of spectators from all sports events was also predicted in a cartoon published in the *Berliner Illustrirten Zeitung* in 1936 (Rürup 1999). Inspired by the near-laboratory preparation and management of the Berlin Olympics the cartoon displayed the start of a sprint races at the Olympics in the year 2000, in a space devoid of any human presence (except for that of the athletes themselves). The starter was replaced by an automatic, electronic apparatus, loudspeakers simulated the cheers of the crowd and a mobile television camera ran along a track, parallel with the athletes, to relay the scene to a domestic audience. Remaining in the world of science fiction, a few years later the application of science in the production of the cyborg body was predicted for Olympic sport in Knud Lundberg's (1958) novel, *The Olympic Hope*. The scientifically synthetic environment became mirrored in the scientifically synthetic body of the athletes.

The gradual territorialisation of spectators has been progressively enforced in British stadiums during the course of this century. From relatively open spaces to enclosed, all-seat stadiums, the sport environment has become increasingly panopticised, subject to an increasing number of hierarchical and disciplinary gazes. Televised sport continues the general trend. The banning of spectators furthers the domestication and the spatial confinement of the spectating experience. In an empty stadium, the world could watch on tv "a pure form of the event from which all passion as been removed" (Baudrillard, 1993). The shape of the future is recalled by Baudrillard in his allusion to a football match between Real Madrid and Naples –a European Cup match in 1987 when the game took place in an empty stadium as a result of disciplinary measures against Madrid from a previous game. This "phantom football match" is described by Baudrillard as

> ... a world where a 'real' event occurs in a vacuum, stripped of its context and visible only from afar, televisually. Here we have a sort of surgically accurate prefigurement of the events of our future: events so minimal that they might well not need to take place at all – along with their maximal enlargement on screens. No one will have directly experienced the actual course of such happenings, but everyone will have received an image of them. A pure event, in other words, devoid of any reference to nature, and readily susceptible to replacement by synthetic images (Baudrillard, 1993).

Television sport produces a sport landscape of sameness. Drawing on the writing of Virilio we can note the difference between spectating at a sports event and watching it on television (Virilio 1991). At a sports event no two people see the same thing (because no two people can occupy exactly the same place) whereas the game on tv is exactly what the camera saw. Spectators see this wherever they sit. Television re-places spectators. More significantly, however, Virilio and Baudrillard draw attention to, and provide the solution to, one of the problems of the sports landscape already alluded to in this chapter – that the intrusion of spectators transforms what should be a sports space into a sporting place – sometimes a sport place of disport. Virilio (1991) notes that the potential exists for the placelessness of sport to become literal – stadiums can be abolished and live performers be replaced with televisual images that would be shown in a video-stadium without sports players, for consumption to tele-spectators. To some extent this already exists: the presence of jumbo-tron video screens inside stadiums, which relay slow motion replays and the fine detail of the action, has become the defining reality for many sports fans –a postmodern condition where the image is superior to the reality.

The one thing that Baudrillard and Virilio do not recognise (or do not make explicit) is that their scenarios would also satisfy perfectly the norms of achievement sport – the "surgical" space in which this event takes place provides the placeless environment insisted on by the achievement and fair play norms of sport. Virilio's prescription that the architecture of sports places "would become no more than the scaffolding for an artificial environment, one whose physical dimensions have become instantaneous opto-electronic information" (Virilio 1991), is a dystopian milieu but one which is predicted by my sport-geographic model.

Epilogue: Three Views of the Same Game

Paradoxically, however, place can be reclaimed from the flat plane of such a televisual dystopia. Let me illustrate the continued contestation of the ideal, pure-space of the normative sports environment by an empirical allusion to the environments of the 1992 European Football Championship final between Denmark and Germany, which was played in the Swedish city of Gothenburg. The game was actually played – and re-(p)layed – in three different (kinds of) places, each of which was a different spectating environment.

The first was the "real" game, being played in Gothenburg. Many thousands of fans witnessed the live game from their individualised, numbered and surveilled cells at he Nya Ullevi Stadium. Although the stadium is a high-tech concrete bowl, there can be little doubt that a strong sense of place was obtained by the huge Danish contingent that crossed the Oresund from Copenhagen. Who is to say that the huge crowd of "Vikings" did not influence the performance (in fact, the victory) of the Danish team, the neutrality of the large number of Swedish spectators being temporarily removed as they supported their Nordic neighbours? Although the space of the stadium was the same as any other, the crowd transformed it into a place of power, passion and of national significance.

The second environment in which the game was (re)played was the homes of the millions of European tele-viewers who watched it. For this huge audience television provided a social context, the way of joining a crowd (Adams 1992). Television can be read as a gathering place; after all, domestically-confined sports fans "experientially inhabit it and relate to other persons through it or with it". It undoubtedly constructs meaningful human experiences. It is not entirely inappropriate that in England pubs that attract clients in part, at least, through the presence of televised sport (advertised to the public as "live"), have been labelled the "new terraces". The same could be said of the US sports bar. Television "draws us in", allows us to cross-experiential boundaries. But television audiences are unable (yet) to influence the outcome of the event they are watching. They are also confined in domestic space in which domestic constraints on behaviour are as rigid – if not more so – than those in the stadium at which the game is "actually" being played. Watching sport in a domestic situation cannot easily be interpreted as a form of resistance – in fact, the exact opposite would seem to be the case. Indeed, as Adams points out, "throwing a brick through a tv screen has not effect on what is seen on any other screen" (Adams, 1992), let alone the course of the game that is being televised. Nor, in a domestic context, would such resistance have any effect outside the domestic cell.

The third environment in which the game was played was conceptually (and geographically) some way between the stadium and the home. In Copenhagen, near the national sport stadium, lies a large area of open space known as Fælled. This area was once common grazing land and was the original locus of Danish football. Today it is a large area of park-land, given over to the playing of club-level soccer. The site has a certain significance to Danes, being the "home" of one of their sporting tradi-tions. On the night of the Denmark-Germany game a huge tv screen was erected in the open space of the Fælled. This was not domesticated tele-vision space in the sense of a small box being in the corner of a living room. It was open, unenclosed and contained no seats. Nor were there any obvious controls on the sale and consumption of alcohol. A vast crowd attended to watch the game. It was mediated by television but the crowd could, for a night, celebrate in the open space. It was a form of carnival with drunken fans celebrating their small nation's victory over the German "machine". Who is to say that the experience of the Fælled was anything but the optimal sporting experience for late modernity – thousands watching in open spaces without being able to influence the game, but standing in opposition to the panopticised confinement that the modern stadium enforces. It was an inconguous juxtapositioning of late-modern and "folk" traditions. In a way, this kind of situation satisfies the norms of achievement sport and also the desires of the fans. It is not quite placeless. It exemplifies a tension between the apparently logical need for a predictable environment and the place-making potential of fandom. It also illustrates the tension between the certain, safe world of "the scientist" and the ambiguous world of "the human" – or the "hard" and "soft" worlds of sport.

References

Adams, P. (1992). 'Television as Gathering Place', *Annals of the Association of American Geographers*, 82, 1, pp. 117-35.

Augé, M. (1995). *Non-Places: Introduction to an Anthology of Modernity*, London, Verso.

Bale, J. (1994). *Landscapes of Modern Sport*, London, Leicester University Press.

Baudrillard, J. (1993). *The Transparency of Evil*, London, Verso.

Gardner, R. (1995). 'On Performance-Enhancing Substances and the Unfair Advantage argument', in W. Morgan & K. Meier (eds.) *Philosophic Enquiry in Sport*, Champaign, Human Kinetics, pp. 222-31.

Guilianotti, R. (1991). 'The Tartan Army in Italy: The Case of the Carivalesque', *Sociolog-ical Review*, 39, 9, pp. 503-27.

Lefebvre, H. (1991). *The Production of Space*, Oxford, Blackwell.

Lundberg, K (1958). *The Olympic Hope*, London, Stanley Paul.

Relph, E. (1976). *Place and Placelessness*, London, Pion.

Rürup, R. (1999). *The Olympic Games and National Socialism*, Berlin, Stiftung Topographie des Terrors.

Sack, R. (1986). *Human Territoriality*, Cambridge, Cambridge University Press.

Schwartz, B. & Barsky, B. (1977) 'The Home Advantage', *Social Forces*, 55, pp. 641-66.

Shore, B. (1995). 'Marginal Play: Sport at the Borderlands of Space and Time', in O. Weiss & W. Schultz (eds.) *Sport in Space and Time*, Vienna, Vienna University Press, pp. 111-25.

Tuan, Y-F (1974). *Topophilia: A Study of Environmental Perception, Attitudes and Values*, Englewood Cliffs, NJ., Prentice Hall.

Virilio, P. (1991). *The Lost Dimension*, New York, Semiotext(e).

Wagner, P. (1981). 'Sport: culture and geography', in A. Pred (ed.), *Space and Time in Geography*, Lund, Gleerup.

Weiss, P. (1968). *Sport: a Philosophic Enquiry*, Carbondale, University of Southern Illinois Press.

Zeller, R.& Jurkovac, T. (1989). 'A Dome Stadium: Does it Help the Home Team in the National Football League?' *Sport Place*, 3, 3, pp. 36-9.

CHAPTER FIVE

Scandalous Sport: Finland as a Case Study

Niels Kayser Nielsen

On Monday 13 November 1893 a big banquet was held in the hall of the Society House in Helsinki, with the purpose of raising money for a new folk high school in South Karelia. A lottery with prizes in the form of donations from the handicraft guilds of the country was therefore part of the banquet. The event was supported further by the leading academic and commercial circles of the city, headed by two brewery kings (Hartwall and Sinebrychoff). The first performance of a work of Jean Sibelius, Karelian Scenic Music, consisting of an overture and a series of tableaux from the history of Karelia, was also part of the banquet. In the first of these tableaux, the setting is a Karelia home in the year 1293. They are having a pleasant time, with ballads (the so-called 'runor') and Finnish national romance. All is quiet and peaceful, until a giant bang sounds! The peace is over. A catastrophe has taken place and the horror is spreading. The enemy has invaded the country (Kvist Dahstedt 1999).

A similar thing happened on 28 February 2001. On that day Finnish ski sport died. What had promised to be a glorious celebration turned into one of the biggest scandals in the history of sports, and definitely the biggest in the history of Finnish sports. The catastrophe is of course the exposure of six Finnish skiers' doping abuse at the Lahti World Championships in cross-country skiing, of whom Jari Isometsä, Harri Kirvesniemi and Mika Myllylä are the best known. As in the Karelian home in 1293 and in the Society House 600 years later, the idyll was perforated. At first disguised as shame and anger; and national indignation, the Finnish people felt outraged by the world of sports, and disorientated: "This is just as unthinkable as if Mannerheim was a 'trans'", the biggest newspaper *Helsingin Sanomat* wrote on 3 March 2001. At the other end of the scale, the popular weekly *Suomen Kuvalehti*, on 2 March 2001, quoted the Chairman of the Finnish Ski Association as stating, "We are poor creatures". In the same weekly, on 9 March, the Finnish President Tarja Halonen said, "There is no doubt that it has compromised the reputation of Finland". There was thus evidence of a nationally significant and public dimension to the affair from the very start. This is hardly odd, since the matter concerned the Finnish heart blood of skiing: "Skiing is still the sport of the Finnish rural population", a comment stated at the time (*Helsingin Sanomat* on 4 March 2001). As we will see below, this is historically correct.

The outrage is to be seen in contrast to the fact that Finnish ski sport receives 4.5 million Marks each year, equivalent to approximately 5.6 million Danish Kroner ($700,000), from the state budget. This amount of money seems poorly spent, now that the scandal of doping, cheating, and fraud has been exposed. Based on a cost/benefit calculation it certainly looks like a bad bargain, not least because the matter appears to be a national Finnish problem. This is, however, not just the case. It is not only Finland that has a problem, but also sport. Or rather – and this is the first hypothesis of the present chapter – sport does not have a problem, but is in itself a problem. This problem will be brought into focus below. But first I will deal with Finnish nationalism and features of the history of Finnish sports. Then I will focus on sport and its nature in relation to the special circumstances in Finland in the hope of casting light on the present situation.

It is often said that sport is apolitical. More reasonable people claim sport to be political; it is said to be influenced by society that penetrates all pores of sport and, as a result, ensures that any purity of sport is nullified. But perhaps it is really the other way around: society is imbued with sport. While some scholars have acknowledged this, it bears repeating in this argument and thus forms the second hypothesis of the chapter.

More specifically, the chapter focuses on the weaving together of sport and society that has worked in the service of nationalism, but which is now disintegrating, partly because nationalism is changing, partly because sport is running amok, and neither bodies nor nationalism can keep up. This has the effect that sport represents a threat to nationalism. With a few detours to the other Nordic countries, the chapter will seek to demonstrate that the relationship between sport and nationalism is a precarious matter, not only in Finland, but anywhere. Who is using whom? one might ask.

Finnish nationalism

Finnish Nationalism is, to a great extent, determined by geopolitical and geographic circumstances, but it also significant that Finland has been part of the Swedish-Finnish realm since the earliest concentrations of power took place in the Middle Ages. The idea of a "pure" Finland and a "pure" Sweden is no more than some hundred years old and can justifiably only be said to apply from 1917 and 1905, respectively – and even here it is problematic to speak of "purity", partly because there is still a large Swedish-speaking population in Finland, partly because a large part of the administrative, juridical, and political practice in Finland is still of Swedish origin. There is an ongoing lively debate both in Finland and in

Sweden about the extent of Swedish origins. It is crucial for the question whether Finland is a Nordic country – or a unique case.

Some Finnish historians and cultural theorists claim that the latter is true. They advocate that through moves towards an independent Finnish 'state', which accelerated after 1809, when Czar Alexander I at Borgå Landdag granted Finland a seat in "the number of nations," Finland's path is unique.

If this viewpoint is valid, it can be added that Finland's nationalism is based on the concept of standing alone in the world and is "only" supported by the internal coherence and trust between state, society and citizens. In other words, no one can fail or let themselves be seduced by foreign non-Finnish forces. Finland has a keen eye for this and it has been so from the beginning of the Finnish national state. This perception of the nation has, on the other hand, always had a keen eye for European influence and has endeavoured to make Finland appear as a modern civilised country – a country "in the swim".

In opposition to the isolationist viewpoint are Max Engman and the Swede Torkel Jansson, who have both advocated the viewpoint that the Swedish heritage has more weight. Engman points to social conditions (a strong and independent peasantry) as well as the legalistic heritage (Engman 1994; 2000b). Jansson also indicates these factors, but further points to the common local administrative heritage in the form of the so-called "*sockenstämmor*", which gave both Sweden and Finland the tradition of a strong local self-government – stronger than in both Denmark and Norway (Jansson 1997a, 1997b, 2000). Both researchers further point to the close semantic linguistic connection between Swedish and Finnish. Other scholars have pointed to the Lutheran-Protestant heritage, which attaches great importance to the responsibility of the individual toward authorities, consensus, and conformity (Stenius 1997).

Max Engman finds that Finland is a Nordic country in the last resort and furthermore that it means that with respect to nationalism Finland has a Nordic position characterised by a hybridisation of a Western European and Eastern European way of forming a nation and a national self-consciousness. This hybrid consists of a mixture of universalistic and particularistic principles. On the one hand you can say that history can become rational if you take departure in certain general principles, among them that human beings are free and equal rational beings. On the other hand, that reason is always historical in so far that it relies on specific local circumstances that can never be disregarded.

This duality is sometimes described as a combination of a political and a cultural nationalism. In the first case, weight is attached to political-voluntaristic principles and the sphere of action of the individual; based on the *ius soli* principle. In the second case, history, language, and cultural heritage are stressed (in some vulgar interpretations also race) on the basis of the *ius sanguinis* principle. In the first case, the voting rights and equal opportunities independent of birth are crucial. In the second case it is not individuals and their rights that are important, but the community and nationality. Here it is not the polling place and the parliament that matter, but instead the games, national festivals, and the cultural rituals for enrolling the individual into an organic whole (Hettne, Sörling, & Østergaard 1998).

It may plausibly be asserted that Nordic nationalism and thus also Finnish is characterised by these principles. This applies to the state nations of Denmark and Sweden, but not so much to the national states Norway, Iceland, and Finland, where there was a national movement before a state. The issue has been quite extensively debated in Norway, in so far that the idea that Norway first had the Eidsvoll constitution and then a Norwegian culture of national independence is also present here. This means a situation like that in Italy, according to d'Azeglio, where there was first an Italy and then Italians. Whether one or the other viewpoint is correct, it is a fact that the history of Norway in the 19th century has been characterised by both a strong democratic conscience (the strongest in the Nordic countries – and sometimes even radical-democratic in its aim) and a strong popular mobilisation from the bottom.

The same applied to Finland but never in a radical-democratic sense. Finnish nationalism was formed by the strong Hegel-inspired Fennoman and etatistic thinking that with a distinct *festina lente* attitude would both solidarise with and educate the population *von oben*. At the same time there was a characteristic dual movement, supporting the special status tolerated by Russia as an independent Grand Duchy and (more or less under coercion) using the Swedish administrative and educational heritage (Klinge 1988: 95 ff.)

The consequence hereof was that the activities targeting a general education of the population, which had been initiated everywhere in Finland in the second half of the 19th century, became constitutional and state-oriented to a marked extent. This state of things is reflected, for example, in the language. It is hardly a coincidence that the Finnish language uses the same word for citizen and nation, i.e. *"kansalainen"*; a word derived of the word *"kansa"*, which means both state, society, people, and nation. As the Norwegian sociologist Dag Østerberg once said, it is impossible to write the history of the Nordic countries without Hegel. This particularly applies to Finland. Here one is both a *citoyen* and a *Volksgenosse* (Engman 2000a: 9). This implied a wide-ranging general education. The people had to be trained to be citizens, which at the same time meant respect for and a reflexive revival of the Finnish people's own traditions and folk culture, or, if you prefer, a combination of modern rationality and traditional idealism (Högnäs 2000: 25). As part of the dual movement, the aim could be to enrol Finland into a European cultural context; the way it took place at the Karelia banquet, where Sibelius' orchestral work had references to both Lutheran psalms and Bach's chorals, and develop distinctive Finnish features (folk songs, traditions, customs, and a certain "Mongolianity") as part in the cultivation of a national and cultural character (Kemiläinen 1998).

Sports could also be used in educational work. This applies whether the emphasis is laid on the etatistic-Fennoman nationalism or the Nordic heritage. Sport could serve both cases since they are occupied with combining both national festivals and the *citoyen* dimension. And in both cases, sport offers its services, partly by showing unison between the nation and the citizen by virtue of the grand and festive performance on behalf of the nation, partly by stressing the element of equality and liberty as the point of departure of sport, respectively. One starts on equal terms and a winner is found in the end; liberalistically. In principle, sports and the national, with respect to both political and cultural nationalism, get along well and can use each other as a lever.

Features of Finnish sports history

National historians have stressed that Finnish sports have been an important co-player in the national revival that took place during the second half of the nineteenth century and up to 1917 and beyond. In the time before independence the earliest history of sport is very often connected to national festivals and lotteries partly for the benefit of Finnish nationalism in general, partly for the building of certain houses and institutions, such as the House of Students in Helsinki. Civil society also took an active part in this process, not only in the capital, but also in the rural districts (Lehtinen 1996). Already in the 1840s, Topelius had realised that sports activities had a class-fraternising effect, and, in the excursions and festivals that were arranged for the town population, competitions soon became an obligatory feature. These competitions further achieved an important legitimacy as they were a useful element in the political struggle for the physical life of the nation. They could be used in the defence of the country. This is illustrated by one of these national festivals, the Fritidsveckan in Helsinki in the 1870s, which has been studied by Henrik Stenius. It is characteristic here that it is to an increasing degree sport, in and of itself, that gains ground. The idealistic and nationalistic element does not disappear, but sport itself is increasingly at the centre of interest (Stenius 1981).

Similarly, a number of studies on the Swedish-Finnish Kammerat-Movement have shown that the festive and enjoyable atmosphere that played such a big role in the first decades of the history of the popular movement is gradually giving in to the strictly sportive (Wikman 1963).

The previously popular combination of social life and sport is dwindling, and at the same time the specialisation of sportspeople increases, so that they concentrate on the practice of one sport exclusively to an increasing extent (Björkman 1997: 19 ff.). The festive element disappears; the competition and its pragmatic lose-or-win code conquers.

The final victory of sportification does, however, not seem to have been won until after a long and tough struggle. Kenth Sjöblom's study of Finland's oldest gymnastics club, Helsingfors Gymnastikklubb, thus shows that within that sport the competitive factor did not replace the tradition for displays, trips, and tours abroad until the 1950s. The result is, however, unambiguous: the club's aversion to the Olympic competition principle could not be upheld in the long run (Sjöblom 2000: 124 ff., 170 ff.).

During the 19th century, a nationalisation took place in parallel with sportification. Where the Norwegians for national reasons could not readily go in for the Swedish Ling gymnastics, the situation was different in Finland, where Swedish Ling gymnastics represented what had been lost by Russian annexation. There was thus, at first, nothing to prevent gymnastics from becoming a national symbol in Finland. This picture was, however, muddled by one particular important factor, namely that the struggle for national independence in Finland was connected with the struggle for language. Finnish national self-consciousness was from about 1860 Fennoman in the way that it also opposed the Swedish-speaking upper class. Like the Danish Grundvigianism, it lacked a formal congruent organisation, but was instead legitimised by pretending to act on behalf of the people (Alapuro 1987; Stenius 1992). In solidarity with the young-Fennoman endeavour, a number of Swedish-speaking families changed their names from Swedish to Finnish (e.g. Forsman was changed to Koskinen, Gallén to Gallén-Kallela, and Gummerus to Pihkala), just as Jean Sibelius, who was actually descended from a Swedish-speaking civil servant's family, applied himself to the creation of Finnish national-romantic musical iconography. Finnish was regarded as the heart of the nation, while Swedish was considered as the stiff shell (Högnäs 1995: 28). This Fennomanism naturally obstructed the chances of adopting Swedish Ling gymnastics as a national symbol. Like Norway, the Finns had to go their own way, with competitive sports as the big victor (Laine 1992).

One should, however, keep in mind that the building of the independent nation of Finland, also in the twentieth century, was of an entirely different nature than the Norwegian partly because it took place later than in Norway, namely at a time when sports had been generally accepted, at least in the cities. In addition, Finland bordered the Soviet Union and sporting developments, as the rest of society, were influenced by Finland's geographical situation.

It lay near at hand to go for skiing as a national symbol like Norway (Christensen 1993), but as a result of the timing for new nation-building, there were now other possibilities in the form of modern sport. Winter sports including cross-country skiing were therefore supplemented in the summer with athletics and the ball game boboll, which Lauri "Tahko" Phikala constructed as a combination of American baseball and rounders. The idea was to propagate the sport in the Finnish quasi-military "Skyddskårsrörelse" and to use it here as part of a military prep school, e.g. as practice for throwing hand-grenades (Seppälä 2000).

For ideological reasons individual sport prospered in Finland. After the national catastrophe of 1918, Finnish land policy was aimed primarily at procuring access to private property for the impecunious rural population. This was partly to prevent a repetition of the revolt of 1918, which was very much due to lack of land (Peltonen 1992), and partly to propagate individualism and a sense of the private in the general population.

That the Soviet "kolkhoz-thinking" was considered as one of the main enemies was not without meaning: individual sport was rated highly in Finland in the politically combustible inter-war period. In the present connection it is appropriate to quote the editor of the periodical of the Danish Gymnastics Clubs, A. Pedersen Dømmestrup, for the following statement in 1920, which bears further evidence of the kinship between the Grundtvigian gymnastics tradition in Denmark and the Fennoman body-cultural heritage:

> In Finland the young people of the country play sports as they do gymnastics here in Denmark. The young Finnish people, in particular in the countryside, practise sports in the evening and in their leisure time, not at the stadium, due to the long distances, but outside the farm, where they have their daily work. (Pedersen Dømmestrup 1920: 291).

Finland's rural character and low level of urbanisation during the inter-war period also contributed to the strength of individual sports. Even in the rural areas people lived more on individual farms than in villages.

Finland's greatest international success occurred in athletics, in particular in disciplines that are particularly suitable for self-practising, such as long-distance running and javelin throwing. If you look at the world records in athletics in 1934, the records in running from five kilometres up, in discus (aggregated for both hands) and in javelin throwing belong to Finns. Measured in world records, Finland in that year was the world's second-best nation after the USA.

Athletics could be used nationally as a demonstration of the vigorous young Finnish nation. Paavo Nurmi became a national icon, until it went wrong, and it turned out that Nurmi was not just national, but also greedy. Swedish athletics circles headed by Sigfred Edström, who was also the chairman of the International Amateur Athletic Federation, had discovered that Nurmi was part of a professional show business. The sport had in other words eaten into not only the festivities around the sport, but also into the national domain. Nurmi did not only run for the sake of Finland, but also for the sake of the show (Halmesvirta & Roiko-Jokela 1997). This was, however, not really an expression of Nurmi's greediness. It was only fair that he was also handsomely paid for his contribution to the event, when the organisers could make a good profit from his participation in competitions. The problem was in other words not Nurmi, but sport.

The incursion of money into sport was not confined to athletics. It also applied to ski sport. Modern ski sport began, not in the countryside, as might be expected, but in the cities. Organised skiing contests first took place in 1889, in Oulu. The initiators were the bourgeoisie of Oulu, who were aware that there were many good skiers among the rural proletariat, who had been skiing all their lives. And what could better make a man of the people compete in ski sport if not monetary prizes? The prize of victory far exceeded a farmhand's yearly pay. Fourty-four year old Aappo Luomajoki, who otherwise lived as a hunter and lumberjack, won the first competition. He participated in the Oulu games several times, but only as long as he had a chance of winning (Heikkinen 2000). Even in small contests, one could make over 100 marks, i.e. half a year's pay (Salmenkylä 2000). When the amateur rules were systematised after 1900, the large monetary prizes disappeared but were replaced with trophies and other artefacts. In some cases the organisers announced the monetary value of the trophies. Furthermore, the amateur rules could be bent somewhat by paying travelling expenses and maintenance allowance, just as many of the skiers could make an additional profit by selling ski wax (Häyrinen 2000). The sport did thus not only eat into festivals and nationalism, but also the amateur aspect. Where the sport went forward, everything else had to give way.

Sport even ate into the war. During World War II sports were practiced industriously. Some clubs were able to stay in a sort of training camp behind the front of Karelia during the Continuation War (Kayser Nielsen 1997). In Karhumäki, also in Karelia, there were contests in athletics, wrestling, boxing, and football (Römpötti 2000), and also at the Karelia Isthmus, there were contests in boboll, volleyball, and orienteering during the Continuation War (Tolvanen 1997). The supreme command enthusiastically supported these activities, which were a welcome chance to get rid of card games and drinking at the front.

After the Second World War, the first Nordic doping scandals emerged. Denmark took the lead with the tragic doping death of the rider Knud Enemark at the Olympic Games in Rome in 1960. Then followed Norwegian and Swedish sportsmen, and finally Finns. On 4 March 2001, *Helsingin Sanomat* listed the twelve Finnish sportsmen who have been found guilty of doping abuse; among them a number of world names. Lasse Virén has been accused of doping, but without proof. On the other hand, Martti Vainio was caught for doping at the Olympic Games in Los Angeles in 1984. The scandal at the Nordic World Championships in Lahti in 2001 completes the picture.

In some countries, where sports do not have the same national loftiness, they do not take such a situation too much to heart. In Finland, however, where sport has so often been used as a national symbol and propagation instrument, the scandal is seen as a violation of the national self-consciousness. The population feels deceived by sport and see themselves as victims of sportive infringement. This equivalence between sport and nationalism has, however, also been attached in Finland.

Disasters and Savings

1999 has rightly been called the annus horribilis of sports. The otherwise praised and recognised world of sports was dragged through the mud, and one affair after the other was exposed. Doping, bribery, greediness, and lust for power were the order of the day. The extent of the scandals is now so wide-ranging that one is beginning to ask whether it is sport itself that is the problem. The surprising aspect of the whole affair is, however, not the exposure of rottenness in sport. The problem lies in a completely different place, namely in the supposed internal logic of sport. Four arguments play the major role in conceptualising sport in crisis.

The first argument is, by and large, that we have to remove the worst aberrations from sport such as corrupt officials and excessive money. The doping rules have to be made more rigorous, and punishments for one or the other offence have to be adopted. Then the sport will again appear as it really is: clean and pure. But there are grounds for suspicion. This whole basic view is in reality grounded on fundamentalism: "back to basics", as it was called in Thatcher's Great Britain. It is not only in Islam that such fundamentalism exists. It is also thriving very well in the world of sports. However, this is a false logic for if you want to forbid doping, eventually you have to forbid sport.

Basically this idea builds on the perception that sport as such is good enough; and as long as you stick to that basic view, the problem will still not be solved. Because at no point do sports reporters and sports leaders ask whether it is in reality the very nature of sport that is infected. The matter is in all simplicity that doping and economic fraud do not emerge from thin air; they are not accidental. It is the first error of self-criticism that it will not admit to the problem.

The second argument is of a more cultural-theoretical nature. It builds on a basic view that says that beneath the flaws and the scandals, there is a healthy and authentic core, a genuine life of sports: "a sound mind in a sound body". It is a classical Western European conception. It builds on the idea of genuineness and originality, regarding the visible world and the actual phenomena as more or less fortunate manifestations of the genuine original core, which should thus be found. This philosophy of genuineness has always thrived together with fundamentalist tendencies. The same is the case in the sports debate, where there are also all sorts of statements claiming that basically sports are occupied with good. If doping is removed, "clean" sports performance and authentic body activity will be found, as if there is such a concept as the authentic body or clean sport. It is more likely that any body is so profoundly influenced by the surrounding society that it makes no sense at all to operate with the concept of "purity". The conception of purity and genuineness is to a pronounced degree contributing to confusion – and it smells badly of the 1930s.

A third position claims that such considerations are really quite irrelevant. Sport does have a value in itself – doping or not. From this position sport can be seen to have an internal logic, an aesthetic and beauty. One might then just as well be liberal, and sports will not worship beauty any less because performers are doped. It means less, for art(ificiality), aesthetics, and dope go well together; just think about rock stars.

The concept of the internal logic of sport has, however, always had a hard time. In a historical perspective, it rather seems that sport has had to be inflated with importance again and again. It has been attributed one and then another good quality. It is said to be good for democracy and nationalism – and for internationalism. It is also said to have fine character-building properties. To play sports is to train oneself in social consciousness, etc, etc. Thanks to its officious lobbying and others' wishful thinking, sport has been able to secure a legitimacy that is absolutely unheard of in society. Despite the fact that good fellowship is thriving just as well in a choir and an amateur musical club as in a handball club, it is sports and not amateur music that has harvested legitimacy and monetary support.

Finally, there is a fourth argument to the effect that only elite sports are infected. There can, however, be no getting around the facts so easily. Not only at elite level, but right down to the junior ranks and way into the so-called amateur sports, live greediness and a fixation with money. There are nice stories about clubs that pay the junior players pocket money so that they do not have to work; about boys who in winter drive from hall to hall to play indoor football to win prizes in the form of expensive sports suits, which they then sell to the poor creatures who did not win.

A couple of years ago there was a story in the Danish press about a prominent sports leader who had once met the Swedish author and playwright, Per-Olov Enquist. To his great disappointment the sports leader had to acknowledge that Enquist was not particularly interested in discussing sports with him. The leader was almost offended, since Enquist had in fact written both a novel about sports and covered the Olympic Games in Munich. Surely there is no reason for sulking. The matter is most likely just that Enquist did not find sports very interesting, and that being a Swedish champion in high jump, he knew sports from within. In any case his novel *Sekonden* is about what is also the crux of the matter today: that the misery of sports comes from within.

The price for that is now being paid. If the ideals had not been so highly rated, the fall would not have reverberated so loudly. As Ivar Lo-Johansson wrote in 1931, "I have doubts about sports". The world of sports should do the same. But it cannot, because then it will dig its own grave. The doubts concerning the aberrations of sports eventually dispute the very nature of sport.

The "nature" of sport

None of these concepts seem to relate to two of the most central features of sports, namely its 'adaptability' and 'expansionism'. The first feature is attached to the idea of the freedom of value in sports. Sport can without scruples enter into an alliance with any kind of political system: ranging from laissez-faire capitalism over Nordic social-liberal communities to totalitarian regimes such Hitler's Germany and Stalin's Soviet Union. In neither of these latter cases did sport stand back, and in neither case did sport offer serious political or structural resistance. The spinelessness of sport is particularly obvious here. Its simple win-and-lose code can be used everywhere. Sport eats into anything and anybody; and it is not uninteresting to ask oneself the question about the Olympic Games in Berlin in 1936: who really tricked whom? Was it not Hitler's technically perfect framework with a TV inside the Olympic arena that guaranteed sport glamour and legitimacy? Or was it the other way round: that sport guaranteed Hitler glamour and a opportunity to show the world what he could provide? Was it the contrast to the obvious and vulgar willed abuse of sport that opened up the conception of the 'purity' of sport? And did Hitler's and sport's gigantism, in fact, not fit perfectly together? This reasoning does not seem out of line, considering the other feature of sport.

This other feature is the desire for expansion. Citius, altius, fortius is not just about sports competition as such. It cannot be separated from the big system of sports: the alliance between sports economics, sports journalism, and media and sports medicine. The system of sports itself rests on the same base as sports competition. You have to hunt high and low for examples of the fact that the sports system has refrained from expansion. In its innermost presence sport is imperialistic. Slowly but steadily, it eats into increasingly larger parts of social life. A look at the extent of the coverage of sports events in the daily press and the press in general will serve to illustrate the development. Starting from scratch around 1900, the situation is today that sports news clears the front pages daily. The same applies to the visual media. Sports are good television. Very often they are presented in connection with or as part of the news programmes that are considered as the epitome of public service.

Some years ago it was feared that the large commercial TV-companies would conquer sport. One of the most spectacular examples is the story of how Rupert Murdoch's Sky tried to buy Manchester United. The situation has today been replaced by another scenario: sport buying TV companies. The British media consultant William Field from the company Spectrum Strategy Consultancy thus says in an interview in the Danish newspaper *Morgenavisen Jyllands-Posten* that films were the most important product in the media market in the middle of the 1990s. Today it is sports, which can also be communicated through cellular phones. Therefore media companies such as BskyB, Granada, and NTL are present in the boardrooms in approximately half of the British Premier League Clubs. The result has been a tripling of the media income of the Premier League (Brandt 2001). They know how to get value for money and in the long run it is therefore the intention that the clubs themselves transmit their matches through broadband and cellular phones. The monopoly of TV stations is thus under severe pressure. Also here sports are gaining ground.

That TV is in the pocket of sports appears from the transmission of the Swedish Radio TV 1 from the first major skiing competition, i.e. the World Cup Championships in Borlänge on 14 March 2001. The doping case was only mentioned sporadically and briefly. It was only mentioned that the Finnish team had been reduced. There was no debating whether the winner, Sweden's own ski star, Per Olofsson, was doped. The latter can be said to be national sacrilege and the hush-up in the Finland matter could be due to fraternal love. This is, however, a dubious argument, considering the Nurmi case. In the world of sports there is no love.

Closing remarks

The six Finnish skiers ended up in this circus. As marionettes or as 'mortal engines', as John Hoberman calls it, and with devastating consequences. As it says above, Finnish nationalism – whether Fennoman etatistic or Nordic social-liberal oriented – is a suitable battlefield for sports. But while the sport/nationalism cocktail is precious to the Finns, it is also dangerous. They are seriously playing with fire. In 1917 the Finn Artur Eklund published the book *The Philosophy of Sport*. In this book it goes that England is a country so rich and modern that it can refrain from participating in the general enthusiasm for the Olympic palms of victory. In his opinion Finland cannot afford the same, "Our country is small and unnoticed, and we must take every means to further her position; to consolidate her position in the consciousness of the big wide world" (Eklund 1970: 126). He then writes that the runner Hannes Kolehmainen more than anything has put Finland on the map of the world. If Eklund had lived long enough, he could also have mentioned Nurmi and Viren and the skiers in the 1930s and 1950s. He could also have mentioned the pride in hosting the Olympic Games in Helsinki in 1952, when the last indemnity to the Soviet Union was being paid. But had he lived even longer, he would also have witnessed how the balloon of sport and nationalism burst in 2001. Now he can only turn in his grave.

Finland's calamity of sports is that the expectations of most Finns in all sports is so great that sports has become a predator in society; a predator that eats anything and anybody. The Finnish nation now has to pay for it. One could have wished it a better fate. There is now the risk that eighty years of hard work is completely wasted, unless one finds that sport is just sport. But that would probably be too naive.

References

Alapuro, Risto (1987). "De intellektuella, staten och nationen" in: *Historisk Tidsskrift för Finland* vol. 72.

Brandt, Henrik B. (2001). "Fodbold i en ny boldgade" in: *Morgenavisen Jylland-Posten* 28. 2. 2001.

Björkman, Ingmar (1997). *Idrottsföreningen Kamraterna r. f. 100 år för Finlands idrott.* Helsingfors.

Christensen, Olav (1993). *Skiidrett før Sindre. Vinterveien til et nasjonalt selvbilde.* Oslo: Ad Notam Gyldendal

Eklund, Artur (1970). *Idrottens filosofi.* Helsingfors: Söderström.

Engman, Max (1994). "Är Finland ett nordiskt land?" in: *Den jyske Historiker* nr. 69-70.

Engman; Max (2000a). "Folket – en inledning" in: Derek Fewster (ed.): *Folket. Studier i olika vetenskapers syn på begreppet folk.* Helsingfors: Svenska litteratursällskapet.

Engman, Max (2000b). "Historikerna folk" in: Derek Fewster (ed.): *Folket. Studier i olika vetenskapers syn på begreppet folk.* Helsingfors: Svenska litteratursällskapet.

Halmesvirta, Anssi and Heikki Roiko-Jokela (eds.) (1997). "Se toinen Paavo Nurmi – ja varjoon jääneet" in *Finlands idrottshistoriska förenings årsbok* 1997. Helsingfors.

Heikkinen, Antero (2000). "Professionella i spåret" in: Finlands idrottsmuseumsstiftelse (udg.): *Glimtar ur Finlands idrott.* Helsingfors.

Helsingin Sanomat 2. 3. og 4. 3. 2001

Hettne, Björn, Sverker Sörlin and Uffe Østergård (1998). *Den globala nationalismen. Nationalstatens historia och framtid.* Stockhom: SNS.

Häyrinen, Reijo (2000). "Tävlingsidrottens genombrott" in: Finlands idrottsmuseumsstiftelse (udg.): *Glimtar ur Finlands idrott.* Helsingfors.

Högnäs, Sten (1995). *Kustens och skogarnas folk. Om synen på svenskt och finskt lynne.* Stockholm: Atlantis.

Högnäs, Sten (2000). ""Rika malmådror av ädel metall". Folket som resurs", in: Derek Fewster (ed.): *Folket. Studier i olika vetenskapers syn på begreppet folk.* Helsingfors: Svenska litteratursällskapet.

Jansson, Torkel (1997a). "Nationella, regionala och lokala aspekter på nationsbygget i Norden", in: Maria Fremer, Pirkko Lilius og Mirja Saari (eds.): *Norden i Europa. Brott eller kontinuitet?*. Helsingfors: Institutionen för nordiska språk och nordisk litteratur.

Jansson, Torkel (1997b) "To riger bliver til fem nationalstater – og flere nationer" in: Henrik S. Nissen (ed.): *Nordens historie 1397-1997. 10 essays*. København: DRMultimedie.

Jansson, Torkel (2000). "Två stater – en kultur. Sverige och Finland efter 1809" in: *Historisk Tidskrift – Sverige* 2000: 4.

Kayser Nielsen Niels (1997). "Idræt ved fronten – fra uorganiseret til organiseret idræt i Finland under og efter 2. verdenskrig" in: Jørn Hansen (ed.): *Idrætshistorisk Årbog* (1996).

Kemiläinen, Aira (1998). *Finns in the Shadow of the "Aryans". Race Theories and Racism*: Helsingfors: SHS.

Klinge, Matti (1988). *Från lojalism till rysshat*. Helsingfors: Söderström.

Klinge, Matti (1996). *Finlands historia* bd. 3. Helsingfors: Schildts.

Kvist Dahlstedt, Barbro (1999). "Nationell hängivenhet. Sibelis Kareliamusik och den vesteuropeiska identiteten i 1890-talets Finland" in: Barbro Kvist Dahlstedt and Sten Dahlstedt (eds.): *Nationell hängivenhet och europeisk klarhet*. Stockholm/Stehag: Brutus Östlings förlag.

Laine, Leena (1992). "Urheilu valtaa mielet" in: Teijo Pyykkönen (ed.): *Suomi uskoi urheiluun. Suomen urheilun ja liikunnan historia. Liikuntatieteellisen Seuran julkaisu* nrr. 131. Helsingfors: VAPK-Kustannus.

Lehtinen, Eeva-Liisa (1996). "Fund-raising Entertainment in Rural Finland During the Nineteenth Century" in: *Scandinavian Journal of History* vol. 21, nr. 4 .

Olin, Kalevi and Matti Penttilä (1994). "Professional Sports Migration to Finland during the 1980s" in: John Bale and Joseph Maguire (eds.): *The Global Sports Arena. Athletic Talent Migration in an Independant World*. London: Frank Cass.

Peltonen, Matti (1992). *Talolliset ja torpparit. Vuosisadan vaihteen maatalouskysymys Suomessa*. Helsingfors: SHS.

Pedersen Dømmestrup, A. (1930) "Idræt!" in: *Dansk Ungdom og Idræt* 1930, nr. 28.

Römpötti, Kalevi (2000). "Frontidrottens höjdpunkt – Karhumäkispelen" in: Finlands idrottsmuseumsstiftelse (udg.): *Glimtar ur Finlands idrott*. Helsingfors.

Salmenkylä, Matti (2000). "Finländska storskidare" in: Finlands idrottsmuseumsstiftelse (udg.): *Glimtar ur Finlands idrott*. Helsingfors.

Seppälä, Raimo (2000). "Lauri "Tahko" Pihkala – en nationell profet" in: Finlands idrottsmuseumsstiftelse (udg.): *Glimtar ur Finlands idrott*. Helsingfors.

Sjöblom, Kenth (2000). *Hälsa, glädje, kamratskap. Helsingfors Gymnastikklubb 1875-1900*. Helsingfors: Helsingfors Gymnastikklubb.

Stenius, Henrik (1981). "Fritidsveckan i Helsingfors på 1870-talet" in: Max Engman et. al. (eds.): *My darling Clio. Vänskrift till Jerker A. Eriksson 22. 10 81*. Helsingfors.

Stenius, Henrik (1992). "Finskhetsrörelsens historia fortfarande oskriven", in: *Historisk Tidskrift för Finland*, vol 77.

Stenius, Henrik (1997). "The Good Life is a Life of Conformity: The Impact of the Lutheran Tradition on Nordic Political Culture" in: Øystein Sørensen og Bo Stråth (eds.): *The Cultural Construction of Norden*. Oslo: Scandinavian University Press.

Suomen Kuvalehti 2001 nr. 9 og 10.

Tolvanen, Ville (1997). "Kilpailua ja kannustamista – miten Karjalan kannaksen joukot urheilivat asemasodan aikana" in: Anssi Halmesvirta and Heikki Roiko-Jokela (eds.): *Se toinen Paavo Nurmi – ja varjoon jääneet. Finlands idrottshistoriska förenings årsbok* 1997. Helsingfors.

Wikman, K. Rob. V. (1963). *Harry Schaumann*. Vasa: Svensk-österbottniska Samfundet.

Translation: Helle O. Andersen

"A Pharmacy on Wheels": Doping and Community Cohesion Among Professional Cyclists Following the Tour de France Scandal of 1998

John Hoberman

When the Tour de France came under attack during the 1998 doping scandal, its organizers, team managers, and athletes reacted to this political and media assault as a community that was bent on defending its autonomy, its values and, not least, its survival as a profitable business operation. The president of the International Cycling Federation (UCI), Hein Verbruggen, expressed his amazement at these events along with an evident resentment directed at certain members of his community who were speaking out about the doping subculture of professional cycling: "I was very shocked when I discovered what Festina was doing," he said "If that sort of thing were the rule, I would resign immediately. But I don't trust these pseudo-doctors and frustrated former riders, who claim that the whole team is 'involved.'"[1] Verbruggen's anger was understandable. The sudden enforcement of a 1989 French anti-doping law had placed the UCI at the epicenter of the greatest doping scandal in the history of sport. What the French police found had demonstrated literally overnight that a leading team was engaged in systematic doping, and that the UCI's doping controls were useless or even fraudulent, depending on how one viewed the integrity of its officials. Three years later, following a massive Italian police raid on riders' hotel rooms during the 2001 Giro d'Italia, Verbruggen adopted the same position in defense of the cycling community. Just as in 1998, he expressed his understanding of the riders' protest action against the enforcers of the law who, once again, had found substantial quantities of illegal performance-enhancing drugs.[2] "I can understand why the riders feel insulted," he said.[3] Defying the world's disapproval, the leader and his rank and file declared that the forces of law and order had invaded and defamed an honorable brotherhood. Possessing its own ideal of ethical behaviour, this hardy fraternity had earned, if not respectability, then at least the right to be left alone.

This essay examines the professional cycling community as the extraordinary social phenomenon it was throughout much of the twentieth

century – a celebrated subculture whose drug-taking was quietly tolerated, as political authorities and the general public chose not to address
the consumption of drugs within this milieu. This immunity to public
disapproval and prosecution occurred within a modern civilization whose
pharmacological mores can seem both arbitrary and hypocritical, and the
tolerated drug culture of the Tour should be seen in this context. If the
Tour has enjoyed a special status as a drug-consuming subculture, there
are reasons this was so. Despite the existence of anti-doping laws dating
from 1965, French society did not prosecute cyclists who were, after all,
French heroes, the "giants of the road". It would appear that the authorities who might have prosecuted drug-taking cyclists had concluded that
the social benefits of doping among cyclists outweighed its costs to
society-at-large. Examining the exceptional status of this group should,
therefore, illuminate important questions about modern feelings concerning the use of performance-enhancing drugs and those who take
them. The history of the Tour makes it clear, for example, that public
opinion about doping does not always conform to the prohibitionist line
that is publicly embraced by most sports officials, and this in itself is a
matter of real social significance. This tacit acceptance of certain kinds of
doping by ordinary people would certainly help to account for inaction
on the part of public prosecutors.

In this essay, however, our central aim is to study the Tour riders as a
drug culture that, during the summer of 1998, suffered a traumatic shock
at the hands of outsiders. One German reporter described the consequences of this assault in the following terms: "Now the bubble has
burst. And the closed society has been exploded. There is not much in the
way of solidarity here. In the last analysis, it's all about money and success."[4] The purpose of this essay is to determine whether or not this is an
accurate assessment. In which ways was this a closed society? Did it (and
does it still) lack real solidarity among its athletes and officials? To what
extent has it "exploded" as a result of the Tour scandal of 1998? And,
finally, to what degree did doping serve to create and then, perhaps,
destroy a "closed" community?

This essay will argue *inter alia* that the solidarity of the professional
cycling fraternity has accommodated the clandestine (but only semi-con-
cealed) consumption of illicit drugs. Solidarity of this kind raises a
number of questions about the sources and the resiliency of group cohesion. What kind of solidarity among athletes can be built upon a shared
allegiance to a clandestine drug culture? What are the other values or
shared experiences that make solidarity possible? Is this a genuine community that can inspire loyalty and self-sacrifice, or is it essentially an
aggregation of individual entrepreneurs who have merely consented to
maintain a mutually advantageous arrangement?

Professional cycling is a closed society for a variety of reasons that are not always associated with the use of illicit drugs. Cycling is a very hard way of life, both physically and mentally, and its hardships certainly create bonds of sympathy and respect between some riders that can exist independent of the doping practices that may also bind them together. Tensions between the sense of honour that many share and the rule-breaking required by doping can create a kind of cognitive dissonance that contributes to separating this guild from the world-at-large. "They all live in a state of schizophrenia," a German sportswriter commented in 2001, "caught between the invocation of a safe and intact world of blameless athletes and the fact that they sometimes get in trouble."[5] This estrangement from how most of the world thinks creates feelings of defiance that are sometimes articulated in public even if they are more likely to indict than exonerate the speaker. For example, after more than two years of denying his drug use following the 1998 scandal, the temperamental French rider Richard Virenque finally confessed at his trial in October 2000. On this occasion, he made a point of emphasizing both the exclusivity that characterizes the brotherhood of riders and the rhetorical devices that are employed to preserve its privacy. "You can't understand, you're not part of the scene; in cycling, you don't say 'doping'," Virenque explained to the ignorant outsiders he was addressing.[6]

The same defiant attitude was heard during the Tour scandal from the director of the Tour, Jean-Marie Leblanc, as he responded to the view that the race should be called off. "We want the Tour, the riders want the Tour, and the spectators to whom we are obligated want it to go on. Even if the intellectuals in Paris may not understand," he commented acerbically.[7] Here the insider invokes both the exclusivity of the fraternity and its relationship to a largely supportive public audience. Three weeks earlier, just after the scandal erupted, Leblanc had sounded the same confident note: "Ten days from now in the Pyrenees, there will be as many spectators as ever. The admirable performances will prevail over everything else."[8] The Tour, he said several days later, "will quickly extricate itself from history."[9] While this sense of the Tour's sovereign autonomy vis-à-vis society-at-large proved to be somewhat unrealistic, the confidence of the Tour director was not entirely misplaced. As the Danish sports scholar Verner Møller pointed out after the Tour scandal: "The opponents of doping simply could not grasp that the revelations and the scandalizing media coverage during the summer of 1998 did not cause the cycling public to turn its back on the event. Given that the whole thing was presented as cheating and fraud, the Tour route should have been wholly depopulated when the riders passed by. But it was not. On the contrary, the public was eager to demonstrate its sympathy and offer its support to the embattled field. It was obvious that these people did not feel cheated."[10] A year later, the German sportswriter Ludger Schulze reported during the 1999 Tour that there was no evidence of a decline in public support. As in previous years, about 15,000,000 people were expected to line the course. "Among cycling fans," he wrote, "doping is an annoying distraction, a minor offence comparable to violating the local speed limit."[11] Indeed, one of the ironies of the "closed" professional cycling culture is its openness to the fans, in that its survival depends on its compact with an enormous and faithful public that values the spectacle more than it seems to care about doping. So an essential element of the Tour riders' claim to their exclusive subculture is the populism that sustains it as a popular cult and commercial enterprise.

One sign of a closed society is its intolerance of dissent, and in this sense the cycling community is no exception. Among the most resented commentators were sports physicians who alleged the existence of widespread doping during the early phase of the Tour scandal, at a time when officials were still denying that doping was a systemic problem among the riders. The UCI-president's slap at "pseudo-doctors and frustrated former riders" just after the 1998 scandal erupted is a case in point. One physician who spoke out was the Swiss sports physician Gerald Gremion: "I estimate that in cycling between 80 and 90 percent of all professionals take doping drugs," he said in August 1998. "I personally doubt that anyone can win the Tour de France today unless he is doped."[12] Two weeks earlier Gremion had asserted that 99 per cent of the riders were doped, an estimate that the Telekom team doctor, Lothar Heinrich, called "a nonsensical statement." The manager of the Mapei team, Patrick Lefevre, called Gremion "a frustrated doctor without a team."[13] Such *ad hominem* attacks, and their implicit critique of the dissidents' motives, are conspicuous among the comments directed against the few anti-doping activists who are associated with professional cycling.

Similar scorn was directed at riders who had complained about doping. "Always the same spokemen, riders who have fallen apart during the Tour," said the Telekom rider Rolf Aldag during the 1998 scandal, clearly implying that ethics was a preoccupation for losers.[14] The most bitterly resented figure of this kind, the French rider Christophe Bassons, came to public attention during the 1999 Tour. Thirteen days into the race, Bassons dropped out on account of "emotional exhaustion". "I felt completely alone," he said. "Hardly anyone would talk to me," including his own teammates. Bassons' personal crusade against doping included a newspaper column that provoked scornful comments about "the journalist", a profession that is considered wholly incompatible with the cyclist's vocation and its vow of silence regarding drugs. As the only rider who would talk publicly about doping during the 1999 Tour, Bassons was targeted by the eventual winner of the race, Lance Armstrong. At one point, Armstrong rode up alongside Bassons and asked him why he was making himself so conspicuous. He should be more careful about what he said, Armstrong warned, since public statements about drugs could hurt his career. "I'm thinking less about myself than about the next gene-ration," Bassons replied. Why not just leave the peloton, Armstrong sug-gested. "I'm not going to do that until I've tried to change cycling," Bas-sons replied. "If Bassons thinks cycling works that way," Armstrong is reported to have said, "he's kidding himself. So he might as well go home." When Jean-Marie Leblanc was asked about Bassons" withdrawal, he called it a case of "suicide."[15] Public moralists were not what cycling needed in its hour of peril. Cynical hyperbole of this kind belongs, as we shall see, to a larger repertory of rhetorical strategies that is intended to preserve the closed character of the cycling fraternity.

The offense committed by a dissident such as Bassons is his refusal to conform to what many members of the cycling subculture regard as a utilitarian doping regimen that is no one's business but their own. (The German sportswriter Thomas Kistner has called this consensual cover-up "the silence of the lemmings".[16]) Doping of this kind is not comparable to the pursuit of intoxication by means of "recreational" drugs, and in one sense, some riders claim, it is not even voluntary. "No one starts out wanting to dope," one rider told the Irish sportswriter David Walsh, "but you become a victim of the sport."[17] This process was described by the Swiss rider Alex Zülle after his arrest and interrogation by French police in July 1998: "I've been in this business for a long time. I know what goes on. And not just me, everyone knows: The riders, the team leaders, the organizers, the officials, the journalists. As a rider you feel tied into this system. It's like being on the highway. The law says there's a speed limit of 65, but everyone is driving 70 or faster. Why should I be the one who obeys the speed limit? So I had two alternatives: either fit in and go along with the others or go back to being a house painter. And who in my situ-ation would have done that?"[18] The fact that Zülle's public comments did not make him a pariah within the cycling community showed that the community regarded his motives to be more important than what he actually said. Everyone understood that Zülle had been traumatized by his ordeal at the hands of the French police, and it was this circumstance that allowed him to retain his citizenship within the community.[19]

Resentful insiders may see the dissident's objections to doping as a form of shallow moralizing that expresses a self-righteous exhibitionism rather than convictions that command respect. This position was adopted by UCI-president Hein Verbruggen in January 2000 in the wake of doping confessions by three Dutch riders: Steven Rooks, Maarten Du-crot and Peter Winnen. The UCI-chief simply dismissed their claim that they had been prompted by ethical considerations: "With their confes-sion, they have created an impression that doping was endemic inside their teams and that they had no other option. That is complete non-sense. A rider always bears the primary responsibility for doping. They could have said: 'We're not going to do it'. I have no respect for them."[20] Verbruggen's disdain is unconvincing because it ignores the economic facts of life he has acknowledged on other occasions, namely, the fact that riders are workers who do not want to lose their jobs and who may well sue their federation to keep them. That is why the UCI opposed the two-year doping ban proposed by the International Olympic Committee (IOC) at its World Antidoping Conference in February 1999. The job security of professional athletes, according to this view, should not be contingent on their demonstrated abstinence from work-related drug use. At the same time, this sort of pragmatism does not accommodate ethical objections to doping, which are regarded as a gratuitous kind of nest-fouling that endangers the community as a whole.

The same determination to impugn a dissident's motives seems to have prompted Lance Armstrong's approach to Christophe Bassons in 1999. Such attacks are sincere in the sense that the rider who adheres to the law of silence may not believe that doping is wrong. In one of his less defensive moments, Jean-Marie Leblanc, himself a former professional cyclist, explained the psychology of this world-view. "I am convinced," he said, "that the vice [of doping] is inherent in the practice of elite cycling. Why? Because much of a rider's behavior involves bluffing his opponent, getting him into difficulty, exposing him to the wind . . . in a word, fooling him! By a kind of natural extension, certain riders are inclined to see doping as a permissible strategy."[21] This sort of candor, like that of Alex Zülle, exemplifies the ethical twilight zone in which professional cycling exists, where admissions of doping emerge only in unguarded moments, when riders are under pressure, or when they simply feel like unburdening themselves to outsiders.

The cycling community has accepted episodic public candor about doping for many years, but on the condition that the rider who speaks out does not harbour reformist ambitions in the manner of Bassons. In 1969, for example, one of the greatest of the modern professional cyclists, Jacques Anquetil, a five-time Tour de France champion, said the following in an interview: "I dope myself. Everyone [that is, everyone who is a competitive cyclist] dopes himself. Obviously, we can do without them in a race, but then we will pedal 15 miles an hour [instead of 25]. Since we are constantly asked to go faster and to make ever greater efforts, we are obliged to take stimulants."[22] "People talk so much about doping," the West German rider Dietrich Thurau said in 1977. "But if you don't take anything these days, then you're not going to get anywhere."[23] Such revelations do not scandalize professional cyclists because they do not threaten the consensus that normalizes doping. On the contrary, they offer a blunt and unapologetic explanation of how doping sustains the spectacle the sporting public demands. This rationale for doping points in turn to the professional status of these athletes and their unstated right as labourers to the drugs that allow them to keep their jobs. For it is the right to work, not the ethics of amateur sport, that prevails in the minds of these worker-athletes.

Candor of this kind is less common, however, than the lies and evasive rhetorical formulas the cycling community has employed to conceal the doping subculture from public scrutiny. This repertory of verbal techniques was on full display during the early phase of the Tour scandal. Caught off-guard and confronted by packs of insatiable reporters, cycling officials and riders improvised furiously at impromptu press conferences, groping for verbal formulas that would avoid outright lying while expressing their outraged sense of having been violated and betrayed by people and circumstances that had spun out of control. Jean-Marie Leblanc, general director of the Société du Tour de France, offered a solemn statement of principle: "It is a question of credibility and ethics," he said only days after the scandal broke. "The Tour must remain clean."[24] The fact that the Tour had not been "clean" for decades was lost in the Orwellian mendacity of Leblanc's suggestion that it could be rescued from a handful of scoundrels and be restored to its previously drug-free state. Representatives of the Festina team told one lie after the next. "Our success has nothing to do with doping," said the Festina manager, Bruno Roussel, whose tell-all memoir would appear three years later.[25] "I'm there to take care of the athletes and their health," said the team's head physician, Eric Ryckaert. "I am against doping. Let justice take its course."[26] But riders such as Laurent Brochard, Didier Rous, Luc Leblanc, and Christophe Bassons told a different story about Ryckaert's attitude toward drugs. According to Brochard and Rous, Ryckaert had assured them that he would never endanger their health. Bassons recalled Ryckaert's warm and persuasive voice and his insistence that he could enable the rider to fulfill his potential by means of erythropoietin (EPO).[27] The Festina rider Richard Virenque directed a bitter diatribe against unspecified persons and alluded to imminent legal retaliation. "The hypocrites have got to shut up and look in the mirror," he said. "We were thrown out of the Tour for no reason whatsoever. You will be hearing from us very soon."[28] In October 2000 Virenque finally admitted that he had been doping at the time of the Tour scandal.

The doping crisis of 1998 also elicited more refined rhetorical tricks aimed at asserting riders' innocence. "It is striking," one observer noted at the time, "that among cyclists hardly anyone says that he never dopes – the commonly used verbal formula is: "I've never tested positive."[29] Riders might also talk about "taking care of themselves" [se soigner], "products" rather than drugs, and "recuperation" rather than a drug cure.[30] "I am completely satisfied with what I can achieve with my own physical ability," said Udo Bölts.[31] Three years later, the irrepressible

Marco Pantani, champion of the 1998 Tour, took this slippery style to its outer limits: "In cycling there is not a culture of doping," he said, "but rather a culture of champions, meaning: self-improvement. That means doing things that are forbidden, but that are only forbidden if they catch you."[32] The sly impudence of this formulation expresses both the cycling community's endemic disdain for doping rules and its special status as a quasi-tolerated doping subculture.

This elliptical style contrasts with the more straightforward mendacity employed by the Italian rider Dario Frigo. Before the 2001 Giro d"Italia, Frigo had held himself up as a model of cycling's drug-free future: "[Gilberto] Simoni and I represent a new generation in cycling, like that of the 1980s before the age of EPO. I have gotten to the top naturally. My performance is based on a willingness to sacrifice and hard training."[33] Alas, when Italian police descended on the riders' hotel rooms in San Remo, on the night of 7 June, they found substantial quantities of doping substances in the rooms of Dario Frigo and others, and he was promptly fired by his team.

In the wake of this new round of negative publicity, the drug-free line was now being adopted by other leading riders, as well. "Whoever tries to dope and gets caught," Jan Ullrich declared, "should not be allowed to come back after one year. He should be permanently banned from cycling." The Deutsche Telekom captain condemned the riders who "take banned drugs and win their races, while the rest of us are trying to get in shape at our normal level of strength and produce good performances."[34] "That is something else that makes me fear for the sport," added Erik Zabel. "That there are still colleagues who cheat and thus risk serious health problems. So I agree with Jan Ullrich, who is calling for strict punishment for these cheaters."[35] The head physician of Ullrich's Telekom team, Lothar Heinrich, spoke as if the psychology of doping were somehow unknown to him: "I don't understand how a rider like Frigo, who is so successful, can take such a risk. I mean a legal as well as a health risk. He's experimenting on himself."[36] Even riders whose doping convictions had made headlines around the world joined in this chorus. Following the Giro d'Italia raids of June 2001, Marco Pantani declared that: "Everything is operating the way it did before. Cycling hasn't changed." Nor would he be surprised, Pantani added, if cycling's hero of the hour, Lance Armstrong turned out to have an elevated hematocrit comparable to his own.[37] By September 2001 the once recalcitrant Richard Virenque was saying that he had detected "a change in attitude" among cyclists, presumably a greater reluctance to dope themselves, and he was bent on making a comeback.[38] It is, of course, difficult to appraise the sincerity of these statements. What we do know is that well-known professional cyclists did not offer public endorsements of these ideals prior to the police raids of 1998.

This cacophony of accusation, indignation and disappointment would appear to contradict the idea that the cycling world constitutes a coherent community built on shared ideals and strategies for survival. For while every community experiences dissension, we may distinguish between two kinds of community. The first is characterized by cooperation, the shared acceptance of principles, and an ethos of restraint on behalf of shared goals. The second type of community is essentially an arrangement, a modus vivendi that allows its members to pursue individual goals in a self-interested way that may well be compatible with community coherence in a functional sense, e.g., the Tour de France as a profitable enterprise. This comparison prompts two fundamental questions about the community of Tour riders: (1) Do they belong to the principled or functional category? and (2) Is it possible for a principled community of athletes to practice doping?

There is much evidence that the cycling world is not a principled community that is governed by an ethos of voluntary cooperation. Yet there are also occasions on which a genuinely fraternal spirit seems to prevail. The resulting ("schizophrenic") predicament of the doping riders is well illustrated by Alex Zülle's account of the position in which he found himself following his arrest in 1998: "When you don't tell the truth right away in this sort of situation, then it becomes more than a white lie. It's not really a matter of your personal self-interest. On the Festina team we had a good team spirit, and nobody wants to wind up being the traitor. You stick together in a very, very difficult situation and you want to hold together as a group."[39] The problem with this sort of solidarity is that it is the product of a siege mentality, and that telling the truth is incompatible with maintaining "a good team spirit". Personal self-interest is subordinated to the law of silence rather than an ideal in which the riders can take pride. The group's involvement with the larger society is evident in that the truth is withheld from outsiders whose intervention is backed by the force of the law. It is thus of sociological significance that "good team spirit" of this kind cannot represent the ideals of a society whose officials have made doping illegal – hence the uncertain status of the post-1998 Tour, which has become an awkward exercise in redemption at the same time that it has remained a popular festival.

A less favorable interpretation of the cycling community's brand of solidarity was offered by the British rider David Millar in 1999: "There are a lot of stupid guys in cycling," he said. "You really have to question whether they have any ethics at all. Before last year's Tour you could understand why people were taking drugs, but since then we've crossed the line. We've got to the point where we can say 'OK, let's stop it'. It's become a moral issue. Before it could be called professionalism, now it's just plain cheating and that's what gets me down."[40] This account suggests that Millar too had accepted doping as an element of "professionalism" prior to the police raids that had transformed doping into a "moral issue" the cycling community had finally had to confront. Yet Millar must also wonder whether his comrades have "any ethics at all". How will they adapt to the brave new world of clean cycling in which Jean-Marie Leblanc must beg them to: "Think about the shame you inflict on your family and friends."[41] In a similar vein, the Italian rider Eric Fottorino describes doping as "a kind of treason, thievery among friends."[42] These comments present a picture that differs from Alex Zülle's account of solidarity under siege, where trust binds together those who share the vow of silence. The alternative scenario, evoked by Millar and Fottorino, is a community fragmented by a climate of mistrust that results from the doping subculture. The instability of this community is thus inseparable from its libertarian pharmacology. As Stephen Roche, the 1987 Tour champion, once put it: "I don't think it's anyone's business other than mine whether I've taken amphetamines or anything else."[43] This is a prescription, not for group solidarity, but for entrepreneurial self-interest. A correlate of this kind of self-determination is the right to physiological privacy. "Publishing the blood values [of the riders] would be a serious violation of personal privacy," says the communication director of the Telekom team, Jürgen Kindervater.[44] But publishing red blood cell counts would also be an essential part of enforcing any anti-doping contract between the riders and a society that has decided in favour of drug-free sport. In the meantime, since 1997 the UCI has been imposing restraint on its clients by disqualifying riders whose red blood cell counts exceed a value that is deemed to be medically safe. This procedure, while tolerating some degree of EPO doping, appears to have succeeded in preventing EPO-related deaths like those of the early 1990s.

The solidarity of the professional cyclists most resembles that of a labour union. In the spring of 1999, just before the "Tour of Redemption", the riders formed an association to represent their interests and elected as its president Francesco Moser, a 47-year-old former rider who declared: "We will not allow ourselves to be criminalized as a group. All doping controls must be carried out under uniform conditions." In electing Moser, the riders chose as their leader a man who admitted he had blood-doped his way to a world record in 1984 and who was now an advocate of regulated doping.[45] "We will have to live with doping," Moser stated in April 1999. "Clean cycling is just an illusion." In the meantime, professional cyclists should be allowed to medicate themselves as they saw fit. "There comes a point where the effects of a drug need to be explained to the rider. If he wants to take it at that point, then let him do it."[46] Once again, the solidarity of the Tour cyclists expressed itself as defiance of drug-free sport. It is also significant that Moser defended doping in terms of a worker's right to medicate himself in response to his working conditions. Similarly, the riders' refusal to proceed after the 1998 and 2001 police raids in France and Italy mimicked, however briefly, strike actions by ordinary workers. As early as 1966, a group of top riders had already demonstrated a kind of labour solidarity by refusing to take drug tests following the professional world road-race championships.[47] A year later, there was "a slowdown strike by cyclists protesting the fact that they were being forced to compete without the aid of their accustomed drugs."[48] It was inevitable, of course, that labour solidarity in defense of drug-taking would eventually come into conflict with an anti-doping morality that derives ultimately from the amateurism of gentlemen.

Once we admit that the athlete is a worker, we must recognize that he may also be a vulnerable or an exploited worker. Keeping one's job, Alex Zülle points out, concerns not only "riders who are making big money, but also family men who are just making a living."[49] "I don't believe that there is even one rider in the field who wants to take drugs," Greg Lemond once said on *Bicyclist Online*. "But half of these guys are high-school drop-outs with a wife and three kids at home; and if they don't deliver the goods, they won't get paid."[50] Such observations make the conflict between professional demands and amateur ideals painfully clear. For the professional rider who survives on the racing circuit, life on the road may be the only realistic alternative to a life of boredom or poverty. This is why the drug-free ideal has not won much of a following among this group. Nor is it surprising that the public that supports the Tour can sympathize with suffering riders who take drugs to make it through the race.[51] The solidarity of the suffering journeymen has an appeal that the solidarity of the spoiled prima donnas does not.

The idea that the professional rider is, in effect, an exploited worker has some influential adherents. "The riders are victims of the system," the French cycling official Daniel Baal said during the 1998 scandal.[52] Three years later Marie-George Buffet, the French minister of youth and sports who supervised the government crackdown that year, stated that: "The doped athlete is above all a victim."[53] In August 1998 she had argued that doping was unethical because it put riders at risk for heart disease, cancer, depression and hepatitis.[54] As a member of the French Communist Party, Buffet regards professional riders as victims of capitalist oppression. In her speech to the Chamber of Deputies on 18 November 1998, she stated that doping was rooted in the relentless pressure [*surenchère*] exerted by "commercial interests" on televised sports. Accelerated competition schedules, overly intensive training regimens, and less time for recuperation created the conditions that led athletes to take drugs.[55] "Riders are individuals who have the right to speak out and refuse to take part in races where there is doping," she declared in 1998.[56] The problem with this position was that, while many of the riders may have shared her view of their vulnerable status, they did not necessarily share her dim view of doping. In fact, Buffet and her forces were greeted, not as liberators, but as oppressors by a professional guild that wanted above all to be left alone. Buffet's anti-doping campaign addressed "a social plague" that was said to threaten the public health. But from the cyclists' standpoint, her error lay in her failure to distinguish between elite athletes and a general public that was not dependent on performance-enhancing drugs to make a living.

This conflict between employment-related doping and official demands for drug-free sport has put cycling officials in a difficult position. On the one hand, UCI-president Verbruggen found himself under pressure from the IOC to adopt strict anti-doping penalties that would mean long periods of unemployment for riders who were caught doping – an initiative he helped to defeat at the World Antidoping Conference in 1999. It is also worth noting that he refused to accept any responsibility for the 1998 Tour scandal that occurred on his watch, despite the fact that UCI doping control had shown itself to be wholly ineffective. A year later Verbruggen made it clear that the entire concept of doping control would have to adapt to the continuing medicalization of high-performance sport: "Society and sport are becoming increasingly adjusted to high-tech medical methods," he said. "It's an irreversible reality. The fight against doping has to adjust to that reality."[57] The UCI regulations adopted in 1999 include a provision that would seem to invite the abuse of hormone therapy by the sort of physician who favours the doping of elite athletes: "Hormone supplementation is acceptable only if it is established that there has occurred an abnormal drop in the hormone level which modern medical knowledge regards as a continuing threat to the health of the athlete."[58] This passage suggests that the UCI shares Marie-George Buffet's concern with the health of professional riders. But the similarity is superficial in that Buffet's public health campaign against hormone doping cannot afford to make concessions to a special interest group such as professional cyclists; she cannot get involved in negotiations about where therapy ends and performance-enhancement begins. Following the first phase of the 1998 crackdown by French police, her public approval rating in France reached an impressive 70 per cent.[59] But it was the federation official who supported his riders through thick and thin, not the crusading government minister, who articulated the economic interests and feelings of this athletic rank and file.

While it is essential to recognize that riders are workers, to depict cycling as merely a labour culture would be a serious distortion of this sport and its storied history. The point here is that journalists and intellectuals have consistently downplayed the labor dimension of the sport in favor of more romantic interpretations of these "giants of the road." Perhaps the best known of these celebrations of the Tour is Roland Barthes' essay "The Tour de France as Epic" (1957). Barthes' interpretation of the Tour emphasizes "the great risk of the ordeal," the "magnificent euphoria" it makes possible, and the mythical essences that animate its colorful cast of characters.[60] At the same time, he points out that the myth of the Tour, the tension between its "vestiges of a very old ethic, feudal or tragic" and "the world of total competition", obscures its commercial core.[61] He does not, however, portray the riders as workers, because this would subvert their status as heroes of an epic ordeal.

Far more problematic than this romanticism is Barthes' treatment of doping – "to dope the racer is as criminal, as sacrilegious as trying to imitate God; it is stealing from God the privilege of the spark."[62] Can it be that this most sophisticated of Parisian intellectuals actually believed that doping was a rare and exotic evil that descended upon riders like an alien curse? At a time when the illicit use of amphetamines pervaded professional cycling, this conception of doping seems improbably naïve. The larger point, however, is that admitting the facts of life about doping would have compromised Barthes' appreciation of "the knightly ethic" and "knightly imperatives" that underlie the dignity of the riders' epic sufferings. For an ordeal governed by ritual creates a world in which riders can achieve a kind of honour amidst the rigors of an almost inhuman competition.

The doping scandals of recent years have threatened a sense of honour that some riders and cycling officials take seriously. For one thing, this unofficial code of conduct makes it possible to claim that the cycling community does amount to something more than an alliance of self-interested entrepreneurs. Invoking – or imposing – this code of honour is also one of the few responses available to the cycling community when doping scandals cast the sport into disrepute. Prior to the 2001 Tour de France, for example, general director Jean-Marie Leblanc convened the riders at a mandatory meeting in Dunkirk and required them to sign a ten-point "Code of Ethics" pertaining to doping.[63] Whether this sort of disciplinary measure amounts to anything more than public relations is a question addressed by this essay, in that it is fair to ask whether the cycling community wants to be "rehabilitated" at all.

As if accusations about drugs were not enough, in his book that came out in June 2001, Bruno Roussel accused Jan Ullrich of having sold a stage victory to Richard Virenque during the 1997 Tour. He also alleged that Virenque and the Danish star Bjarne Riis had taken money to let other riders win races.[64] These accusations provoked responses that called attention to a code of conduct the cycling community was willing to defend in an open and coherent manner.

Bjarne Riis issued a categorical denial that also invoked the idea of an ethical code: "That is complete nonsense. Jan and I entered the Tour to win. If he let Virenque win, that was because he had worked harder during the climb and therefore had a moral right to the victory. I don't believe for a minute that any money changed hands."[65]

Team-Telekom press chief Olaf Ludwig also claimed that the riders' conduct was governed by ethical standards: "It is a tradition in cycling that the rider wearing the yellow jersey gives the day's victory to those who have been riding with him. It's a gentleman's agreement, as when Pantani gave Ullrich the victory on the Col de la Madelaine in 1998, and when Armstrong gave Pantani the victory on Mont Ventoux last year [2000]. But there is no way that money changed hands. Selling victories is not an established practice in cycling."[66] The former Danish rider Brian Holm argued that honoring such gentleman's agreements created a genuine community spirit: "What happens is that the rider wearing the leader's jersey gives the stage victory to one of the rivals who have been sharing the work, and this is one of the unwritten rules of the sport. The race leader is in a good position and can allow himself to give something to others. And he does it, because he knows it creates a kind of sympathy."[67]

While these testimonies appeared to confirm the existence of an ethical code, they also pointed to the closed nature of a community that observes its own rules as well as the sport's reputation as a haven for drugs. "There are those who think that cycling is a corrupt sport," the Danish cycling official Henrik Elmgreen said in June 2001. "We do not feel this way. We think it is a wonderful and fascinating sport that contains a very high degree of justice that has been built into it." If cycling was misunderstood by some outsiders, that was because "its unwritten rules and moral concepts can be difficult to understand for anyone who has not grown up in it or lived one's way into its world. Because there is, of course, a morality and an ethics in cycling, and there are limits one does not cross."[68] In a similar vein, the sympathetic academic cycling fan Verner Møller has argued that "the moral rules that apply within the cycling world differ sharply from those that apply outside it. We are talking here about two cultures with radically different value systems."[69] The unspoken question here is whether the special status of the cycling world entitles its members to an exemption from the War on Drugs.

Those who recognize professional cycling as a unique fraternity may differ on the significance of doping. Hans Wilhelm Gäb, an Opel executive who in 1998 was in charge of distributing $30,000,000 of sports sponsorship money in Germany, paid his respects to professional riders during the Tour scandal by recognizing "the ethos of a group that in the last analysis becomes a conspiratorial community, not through doping, but through a shared adventure in a type of extreme sport." At the same time, Gäb took a hard anti-doping line: "The cheating has long been a part of the system. When the wall of silence came down, the riders got upset, not about the doping, but rather about the investigative methods and the reporting about what was going on." "Only when doping is punished as a dishonest and criminal offence," he said, "is there a chance for a new beginning and that guarantee of equal opportunity which enables sport to survive." But why did doping matter? And why should sport survive? While it is reasonable to assume that Gäb opposed doping as a concerned citizen, he was also representing business interests that were financing elite sport as an investment: "Whoever tolerates doping," he warned, "ruins the image of his company." This unwieldy combination of corporate self-interest and civic-mindedness demanded official action against "the small elite of officials, organizers and riders who discredit sport in general and who are obviously incapable of cleaning up their own operation."[70] From the standpoint of the corporate moralist, professional cyclists were bound to the same rules as everyone else. At the same time, it appeared that he might not have thought through all the implications of "shared adventure in a type of extreme sport."

It is outsiders like Gäb rather than professional cyclists who see riders as adventurers. Despite their willingness to risk life and limb, most professional cyclists tend to be reluctant heroes who are not inclined to dramatize their athletic ordeals. This reticence is probably due in part to the fact that relatively few riders are educated men who have the self-confidence to interpret and dramatize their own lives for other people.[71] It is rather intellectuals and journalists who make the case for the "mythical" stature of these worker-athletes. This division of labour produces in turn divided perspectives on the ordeal that generates the drama. Whereas Laurent Fignon once noted that the French public "likes to see its heroes suffer," the riders themselves do not embrace their suffering with a spectator's essentially aesthetic appreciation of their ordeal.[72] "The sporting public knows the riders' sufferings in all of their forms. They follow the ritual year after year and have found meaning in the sheer energy that is expended, and have learned to appreciate great sacrifices."[73]

The author of these words is the Danish sports critic Verner Møller, who may be counted as a particularly appreciative and insightful spectator of the Tour and its dramas. In his book *The Doping Devil* (1999), Møller defends the autonomy of the professional cycling subculture and its right to practice the self-medication known as doping without interference from outsiders.[74] His argument is that only the members of this subculture are qualified to judge the riders' internal code of behaviour. This heretical position enables Møller to mount a series of challenges to the received wisdom about doping and its allegedly pernicious effects. While all of Møller's arguments deserve careful examination, our task here is to evaluate his position on the nature of the cycling community and its right to use drugs as it sees fit.

Møller argues that professional cyclists legitimate themselves as a community through their shared willingness to engage in medically dangerous behavior that serves the larger society as a cherished spectacle. "The sport would not find itself in a dilemma," he writes, "were it not for the fact that both athletes and their public are drawn to and fascinated by what is extreme and filled with risk." He rejects Marie-George Buffet's claim that the riders are oppressed workers, pointing instead to "the inadequacy of the exploitation thesis as an explanation for why the riders are willing to inflict stress on themselves."[75] Nor does he accept the idea that the cycling community is ethically bankrupt: "The fact that sport does not fulfill ideal conditions does not mean that it lacks ideals."[76] The difficult question that remains is whether this community should be granted the right to use drugs that are banned by other sports.

The key to Møller's analysis is his rejection of the medical argument against doping. The hygienic regulation of high-performance sport is, he says, a contradiction in terms, since elite sport is by its very nature unhealthy.[77] From this perspective, the hygienic paternalism advocated by Buffet and others is misplaced and even absurd: "We still do not understand," he says, "why the athletes are willing to take on the role of the victim, even when this involves taking drugs that may damage their health and are, in the most literal sense, life-threatening."[78] As readers of his book are well aware, Møller is willing to confront a number of difficult issues that sports officials and politicians customarily evade. Here it is the inconsistent regulation of voluntary risk-taking by elite athletes who are subjected to physiological regulation to protect their health, even as they are encouraged to hurtle down mountainsides at 100 kilometers an hour.[79]

This juxtaposition of unequal risks lays bare the essentially libertarian ethos of elite sport that Møller celebrates, and the defense of this shared ethos has played a central role in helping professional cyclists cohere as a community. The French anti-doping campaign of 1998 succeeded in part because it broke open this community by forcing a number of reluctant riders and officials to make politically correct condemnations of doping that violated their own (libertarian) sense of what they were entitled to do with their own bodies.[80] This loss of morale revealed in turn the essential role of the libertarian ethos and the law of silence that had maintained it. For once the riders had been forced to accept this loss of their medical privacy, they found there was no medical doctrine or ethics to replace it. Apart from the candid comments of a few prominent riders like Anquetil, professional cycling had never argued its medical case to the public – the same public that would eventually see riders portrayed in the media as a gang of drug addicts. The riders had never learned how to talk about pain and stress and drugs in an open and honest manner, hence their reliance on the transparent rhetorical trickery described earlier in this essay. By the time Bjarne Riis actually spelled it out on Danish television in August 1998, it was too late to save his reputation and that of his sport.[81]

In summary, the professional cycling community, like most other sports establishments with doping problems, has never confronted the medical costs of high-performance sport in a public forum. This is why the medical care and "doping" of riders degenerated into a tacit conspiracy rather than becoming a health-maintenance operation that could bear the scrutiny of outsiders. The EPO testing inaugurated in March 1997 by the UCI was a late and partial response to the larger health conundrum that persists to this day.

The deeper issue such limited physiological regulation does not address is the physiological severity of the Tour and other long-distance competitions. Here is where the difference between the fraternity of riders and the traditional labour union becomes especially clear. For it is a curious fact that the slow-downs and strikes mounted by cyclists over the past half-century have been directed, not against their extreme suffering and diminished life-spans, but against the regulation of the drugs they use to cope with stress. In fact, the idea of moderating or "humanizing" these competitions has attracted little interest among riders and their physicians. Stress reduction has been endorsed recently by David Millar[82] and the French female champion Jeannie Longo, who has called for "competitions that are on a truly human scale."[83] But this remains a minority opinion that does not even attract the support of doctors, some of whom are resigned to the prevailing stress levels and a medical role that aims at preventing even greater harm to the riders.[84] As the Festina team doctor Daniel Blanc formulated this position in August 1998: "If you want a show you have to protect the athletes, and sometimes the best protection is a little EPO to stabilize the hemoglobin level so they don't get tired and hit by frequent infections. It's better than sending them out to perform these contests of strength in an unprotected state."[85] This "lesser-harm" argument remains the least publicized proposition in modern sports medicine precisely because it is applied at the point where intolerable stress appears to call for banned substances that can provide relief.

The cycling subculture created its own doping predicament many years ago by accepting intolerable stress as the price of staying in business. The medical consequence of this accommodation was a de facto doping culture the cycling community could not defend on principle.[86] While defending doping as an accommodation to the stress of the sport has made sense to many cycling fans, public use of this argument confronts two factors against which it cannot prevail. First, the riders' visible suffering appears to be an essential part of the Tour spectacle, whence Laurent Fignon's wry observation that cycling fans "want to see their heroes suffer."[87] What is more, an open appeal for pain-relieving drugs by the "giants of the road" might well undermine the mystique of the Tour by weakening its association with heroism and martyrdom. Second, this rationale for the use of drugs conflicts with the ethos of a societal War on Drugs that has at times shown little regard for the relief of human suffering.

Finally, is it possible for a principled community of athletes to practice doping? I have argued that a doping culture that operates through peer pressure and secrecy rather than confronting the "inhuman" stress that requires drugs is inherently unstable because it cannot defend its medical interests on principle against outside criticism. One might even argue that professional cyclists essentially abandon their true medical interests by virtue of what they do, leaving each man to fend for himself. In this situation, silence can take on the appearance of solidarity. But as the Tour scandal demonstrated, a refusal to inform on one's peers is an inadequate basis for group cohesion. For once the French police had cracked the wall of silence, confessions and accusations signaled the end of solidarity within this once defiant fraternity. And what had they learned? Only a handful of riders were prepared to say about EPO what a Pentecostal minister in Jamaica recently said about marijuana: "It is not a positive part of our culture. It brings our values down."[88]

Notes

1. "Pseudo-Mediziner," *Süddeutsche Zeitung* (August 7, 1998).
2. "Drogenfahnder stürzen den Giro d"Italia ins Chaos," *Frankfurter Allgemeine Zeitung* (June 8, 2001).
3. "'Operation Glücksklee' begann in verlassenen Hotelzimmern," *Frankfurter Allgemeine Zeitung* (June 9, 2001).
4. "Weiterrollen oder ausreißen," *Süddeutsche Zeitung* (July 31, 1998).
5. "Dope und Spiele," *Süddeutsche Zeitung* (July 7/8, 2001).
6. Jean-François Quénet, *Le procès du dopage: La vérité du jugement* (Paris: Solar, 2001): 30.
7. "'Ich fühle mich wie ein Idiot'," *Süddeutsche Zeitung* (August 3, 1998).
8. "Ein Sprengsatz bedroht die ganze Tour," *Süddeutsche Zeitung* (July 13, 1998).
9. "Unter der Erde, nicht über dem Berg," *Süddeutsche Zeitung* (July 17, 1998).
10. Verner Møller, *Dopingdjævlen – analyse af en hed debat* (Copenhagen: Gyldendal, 1999): 137-138.
11. "Ein Mythos, nach wie vor," *Süddeutsche Zeitung* (July 17/18 1999).
12. ""Ich fühle mich wie ein Idiot"," *Süddeutsche Zeitung* (August 3, 1998).
13. "Die Tour ist vermasselt," *Süddeutsche Zeitung* (July 16, 1998); "Unter der Erde, nicht über dem Berg, *Süddeutsche Zeitung* (July 17, 1998).
14. "Weiterrollen oder ausreißen," *Süddeutsche Zeitung* (July 31, 1998).
15. "Ein Saubermann, verjagt vom Außerirdischen," *Süddeutsche Zeitung* (July 17/18, 2001); "Bassons scheitert an der Mauer des Schweigens," *Süddeutsche Zeitung* (July 19, 2001).
16. "Das Kartell der Heuchler," *Süddeutsche Zeitung* (August 1/2, 1998).
17. David Walsh, "saddled with Suspicion," *Sunday Times* [London] (July 8, 2001)]
18. "Hier sitzen nur Schwerverbrecher," *Süddeutsche Zeitung* (July 27, 1998).
19. "In the beginning," Zülle said, "the officials in Lyons were friendly. But on Thursday evening the horror show began. I was put in an isolation cell and had to strip naked. I

had to give up my belt, shoes, even my glasses. They inspected every body cavity, including my rear end. The night was bad, the bed was dirty and it stank. The next morning they confronted me with the compromising documents they had found. They said that they were used to seeing hardened criminals in the chair I was sitting on. But is that what we are? I wanted out of this hellhole, so I confessed." See "Hier sitzen nur Schwerverbrecher," *Süddeutsche Zeitung* (July 27, 1998).

20. "'Totaler Unsinn'," *Süddeutsche Zeitung* (January 7, 2000).
21. Jean-François Quénet, *Le procès du dopage: La vérité du jugement* (Paris: Solar, 2001): 142.
22. Bil Gilbert, "something on the Ball," *Sports Illustrated* (June 30, 1969): 32.
23. "Intern Dynamit," *Der Spiegel* 27 (June 30, 1980): 183.
24. "Ein Sprengsatz bedroht die ganze Tour," *Süddeutsche Zeitung* (July 13, 1998).
25. "'Ich fühle mich wie ein Idiot'," *Süddeutsche Zeitung* (August 3, 1998).
26. "'Ich fühle mich wie ein Idiot'," *Süddeutsche Zeitung* (August 3, 1998).
27. Jean-François Quénet, *Le procès du dopage: La vérité du jugement* (Paris: Solar, 2001): 47-50.
28. "Sechs neue Festnahmen bei Festina und TVM," *Süddeutsche Zeitung* (July 24, 1998).
29. "Die Scheinheiligkeit der Sport-Funktionäre," *Süddeutsche Zeitung* (July 25/26, 1998).
30. Jean-François Quénet, *Le procès du dopage: La vérité du jugement* (Paris: Solar, 2001): 30, 47.
31. "Ich hätte Tränen in den Augen," *Süddeutsche Zeitung* (August 1/2, 1998).
32. "Pantani verdächtigt Armstrong," *Frankfurter Allgemeine Zeitung* (June 27, 2001).
33. "Ullrich fordert lebenslange Sperre für Dopingsünder," *Frankfurter Allgemeine Zeitung* (June 11, 2001).
34. "Ullrich fordert lebenslange Sperre für Dopingsünder," *Frankfurter Allgemeine Zeitung* (June 11, 2001).
35. "Wettkampfstopp beendet nach neuem Ethik-Kodex," *Frankfurter Allgemeine Zeitung* (June 25, 2001).
36. "Jan Ullrich leidet an Asthma: Seit Jahren mit Kortekoiden behandelt," *Frankfurter Allgemeine Zeitung* (June 12, 2001).
37. "Pantani verdächtigt Armstrong," *Süddeutsche Zeitung* (June 27, 2001).
38. "Ist der Ruf erst ruiniert ...," *Süddeutsche Zeitung* (September 19, 2001).
39. "Hier sitzen nur Schwerverbrecher," *Süddeutsche Zeitung* (July 27, 1998).
40. Andrew Longmore, "Cycling – Time to stop cheating, pleads Millar," *The Independent* (June 27, 1999).
41. "Bei meiner Ehre," *Süddeutsche Zeitung* (July 9, 2001).
42. "En sport fyldt med rullende aftaler," *Politiken* [Copenhagen] (June 21, 2001).
43. Paul Kimmage, *Rough Ride: Behind the Wheel with a Pro Cyclist* (London: Yellow Jersey Press, 1990): xxi.
44. "Transparenz als Problem," *Süddeutsche Zeitung* (June 20, 2001).
45. "Doping-Frust im Reich der Radler," *Süddeutsche Zeitung* (May 17, 1999).
46. "Moser: Doping freigeben," *Süddeutsche Zeitung* (April 10/11, 1999).
47. Tom Donohoe and Neil Johnson, *Foul Play: Drug Abuse in Sports* (Oxford: Basil Blackwell, 1986): 7.
48. Bil Gilbert, "Something Extra on the Ball," *Sports Illustrated* (June 30, 1969): 32.
49. "Hier sitzen nur Schwerverbrecher," *Süddeutsche Zeitung* (July 27, 1998).
50. Quoted in Ulrik Sass, "Dopingdjævlen kan ikke uddrives," *Fyens Stiftstidende* [Denmark] (July 12, 1999).
51. See, for example, Paul Kimmage's commentary on the 1988 Tour de France scandal involving the Spanish rider Pedro Delgado. See *Rough Ride*, 176-178.
52. "Ich fühle mich wie ein Idiot," *Süddeutsche Zeitung* (August 3, 1998).
53. "Voll Härte des Gesetzes," *Der Spiegel* (July 9, 2001).
54. *Le Monde* (August 4, 1998), quoted in *Dopingdjævlen*, 97.

55. The French text appeared on a website whose address I did not record.
56. *Politiken* [Copenhagen] (September 7, 1998), quoted in *Dopingdjævlen*, 187.
57. "Tour's uneasy riders get Tour back on the road," *The Times* [London] (June 29, 1999).
58. Quoted in *Le procès du dopage*, 131.
59. "Madame Buffets zwiespältige Revolution," *Süddeutsche Zeitung* (November 18, 1998).
60. Roland Barthes, "The Tour de France as Epic," in *Mythologies* [1957] (New York: Hill Wang, 1979): 79, 80, 87.
61. "It is in this ambiguity [between "vestiges of a very old ethic, feudal or tragic" and "the world of total competition"] that the essential signification of the Tour consists: the masterly amalgam of the two alibis, idealist and realist, permits the legend to mask perfectly, with a veil at once honorable and exciting, the economic determinisms of our great epic." And: "What is vitiated in the Tour is the basis, the economic motives, the ultimate profit of the ordeal, generator of ideological alibis." See "The Tour de France as Epic," 86, 87-88.
62. "The Tour de France as Epic," 83.
63. "Bei meiner Ehre," *Süddeutsche Zeitung* (July 9, 2001).
64. "Es gibt zwei Zeugen," *Süddeutsche Zeitung* (June 22, 2001); "En sport fyldt med rullende avtaler," *Politiken* (June 21, 2001).
65. "Es gibt zwei Zeugen," *Süddeutsche Zeitung* (June 22, 2001).
66. "Vorwurf der Bestechlichkeit gegen Ullrich," *Süddeutsche Zeitung* (June 21, 2001).
67. "Ære til den ene, penge til den anden," *Politiken* (June 21, 2001).
68. "Du kan ikke købe dig til noget, du ikke er," *Politiken* (June 25, 2001).
69. *Dopingdjævlen*, 92.
70. "Sklaven nützen uns nichts', *Der Spiegel* (August 3, 1998): 94-95.
71. Interviewed in 1989, Laurent Fignon commented: "If I had had better career counseling in school, I wouldn't have decided to become a cyclist." When it was pointed out to him that the French public saw him as an intellectual, Fignon replied: "No, I prefer the image of the adventurer." Nevertheless, this interview makes it clear that Fignon's modesty outweighs his interest in being seen as an "adventurer". See "Ein bißchen wie auf einer Wolke," *Der Spiegel* (July 17, 1989): 172.
72. The interview with Fignon appears in "Ein bißchen wie auf einer Wolke," *Der Spiegel* (July 17, 1989): 172.
73. *Dopingdjævlen*, 111.
74. Møller's work is an essential antidote to the standard anti-doping doctrine that generally ignores the sociological and economic dimensions of the doping phenomenon. At the same time, I do not share his view that the right to practice doping is an inherent part of elite sport. "In our culture," he writes, "doping has become taboo. By violating this taboo – within certain limits – the athletes open a door onto the 'sacred'." See *Dopingdjævlen*, 113.
75. *Dopingdjævlen*, 54, 55.
76. *Dopingdjævlen*, 103.
77. For a more systematic treatment of the problematic relationship between elite sport and good health, see Ivan Waddington, *Sport, Health and Drugs: A Critical Sociological Perspective* (London and New York: E & FN Spon, 2000).
78. *Dopingdjævlen*, 111.
79. See Verner Møller, 'Sport og doping – analyse af en aktuel hysteri," in Jørn Hansen and Niels Grinderslev, eds., *Idræt og samfund, krop og kultur* [*Idrætshistorisk Årbog* 1998, Vol. 14] (Odense: Odense Universitetsforlag, 1999): 152.
80. Møller is surely right to argue that these riders feigned agreement with the anti-doping campaign. See *Dopingdjævlen*, 75; 'Sport og doping – analyse af en aktuel hysteri," 148.

81. "…. I am not saying that we have to practice doping. What I am saying is that we need, one might say, a kind of security. That is why we have doctors with us…." See "Sport og doping – analyse af en aktuel hysteri," 152.

82. "The Tour of Spain is the future of three-week stage races, because they"ve got respect for the riders. If Jean-Marie Leblanc really wants to get rid of doping in cycling, he should take a leaf out of the Tour of Spain's book. The bottom line is that doping exists because racing is so hard. In the Tour, like here, they still race from the gun, but they're doing 200-plus kilometres. Here it's over in three hours. Thanks to the shorter racing time, he [Millar] said, the riders' routine is radically different. "In the Tour it's non-stop before and after the racing as well. Here you get two extra hours sleep per night, you"ve got time to recover." See "The Vuelta the Better," *Cycling Weekly* (October 13, 2001).

83. "Nearing 43, Still at Top Speed," *New York Times* (October 28, 2001). It should be pointed out that Longo has been accused of doping more than once over the course of her long career.

84. Andreas Singler and Gerhard Treutlein have pointed to the striking passivity of high-performance sports physicians for whom the problem of "inhuman" stress during training and competition never seems to be an issue: "One of the remarkable aspects of the physicians' self-image is their constant boasting about their moderating influence, at the same time that they claim to be helpless when confronted with the prevailing [societal] conditions" that demand higher performances. See *Doping – von der Analyse zur Prävention* (Aachen: Meyer & Meyer Verlag, 20001): 40-41.

85. Quoted in "Sport og doping – analyse af en aktuel hysteri," 151.

86. As Ivan Waddington has pointed out: "It is this punishing schedule which largely sustains the tolerance of doping within cycling and, if we are seriously concerned about the health of professional cyclists, then reducing the physical demands made upon cyclists ought to be the first priority." See *Sport, Health and Drugs*, 168.

87. "Ein bißchen wie auf einer Wolke," 172.

88. "Panel Urges Legalization of Marijuana in Jamaica," *New York Times* (September 30, 2001).

Ideal Types and Historical Variation

Allen Guttmann

The first question to be asked about the essence of sports is whether or not it makes any sense at all to ask about the essence of sports. In other words, can the term "sports" be defined precisely enough to refer to all the world's sports in all their historical permutations? Scholars influenced by the Austrian philosopher Ludwig Wittgenstein will counter with the assertion that the search for an "essence of sports" is quixotic and the best we can do in the way of definition is to note a "family resemblance" among a number of related activities.[1] Scholars influenced by the German sociologist Max Weber will answer that there is an "essence of sports" that can be distilled into an "ideal-type" definition.

Since all the contributors to *The Essence of Sport* seem, explicitly or implicitly, to incline toward Weber rather than toward Wittgenstein, an explanation of what Weber means by ideal-type definitions is in order. Definitions of this sort are not meant to be direct statements about the "real world". In Weber's own words, "The more precisely and unambiguously constructed the ideal types are, indeed, the more distant from the real world [*je weltfremder*] they are, the better they fulfill their terminological and classificatory as well as their heuristic functions."[2] Ideal-type definitions are not meant to mirror to empirical reality. They are an abstraction from the disorderly jumble of empirical facts that we stumble upon in our daily lives. They are an attempt to achieve conceptual clarity in order to assess the observed differences between the ideal and the actual.

An acceptance of Weberian ideal-type definitions does not in itself solve any of the empirical problems one faces. If everyone everywhere were to agree on an ideal-type definition of sports, which is fairly unlikely, there would still be disagreement on whether or not various physical activities ought to be considered sports. We might reach a consensus that berry-picking, which was included in a Finnish survey of sports participation,[3] is out of bounds, but there is liable to be disagreement about Formula I automobile races.

What follows is an attempt to (1) formulate an ideal-type definition of sports, (2) relate that statement to the explicit and implicit formulations of the other contributors, and (3) comment on some of the specific issues they discuss. Readers familiar with my previous work (a small group of which I am quite fond) will see that I have revised rather than abandoned the views I expressed in *From Ritual to Record* (1978) and subsequent books. My comments will sound, at times, like *obiter dicta*, but they are merely the best description that I can offer of the paradigm that has, for some thirty years, guided my research into the history of sports.

The key terms in my ideal-type definition of sports are *play, games, contests,* and *sports.* Sports can reasonably be defined as a category of *play* to the degree that they are done for their own sake and not for some utilitarian purpose. As Møller notes, the motivation for sports is intrinsic rather than extrinsic. One becomes involved in a sport – in theory – not for parental approval, academic credit, cardiovascular fitness, or take-home pay, but rather for the intrinsic pleasures of the activity.

The next step in the development of my proposed ideal-type definition is to distinguish between spontaneous and regulated play, between impulsively leaping over a hedge and trying to to leap over the hedge without brushing a leaf. *Games* are regulated play. Since sports are clearly regulated rather than spontaneous play, all sports are games. One of the most fundamental pleasures is that sports take place within a framework of rules that simultaneously enable and constrain. It may seem quirky to refer to gymnastic competitions and track meets as games, but we do, after all, speak of the Olympic Games, ancient and modern. This much linguistic latitude is not too much to ask.

Although many games, like leapfrog and "playing doctor", are non-competitive, other games, like Scrabble and rugby, are *contests* with winners and losers. All sports are contests in which the participants agree to compete against one another, against nature, or against their earlier selves.[4] Competition can be obsessive and excessive, but it cannot be eliminated if a game is to be classified as a sport. The satisfactions of victory and the consolations of defeat are not separable from sports contests as non-utilitarian activities. In fact, the term "sports contest" is redundent because noncompetitive activities are not sports. (Nielsen seems to imply this when he refers to sports "simple win-and-lose code").

If one distinguishes between play and utilitarian effort, between games and spontaneous play, and between contests and noncompetitive games, a fourth distinction follows. The differences between Scrabble and rugby are many, but the most relevant difference for my purpose is clearly that rugby requires much more physical skill. This physical component is what distinguishes some contests as *sports*. To assert this is not to deny that sports also require a mental component, minimal in the case of weightlifting, considerable in most forms of football. There is no *a priori* way to decide how much of a physical component is necessary before a game can be called a sport, but – as a rough test – one can ask whether or not a move can be executed by someone who is not a participant in the game. Poker and chess are not sports because physically disabled players can ask others to hold their cards or move their pawns. Shuffleboard does not require a great deal of physical effort, but octogenerians are required to propel the puck on their own.

Siding with Weber rather than with Wittgenstein leads me to an ideal-type definition of sports – non-utilitarian physical contests – that can be expressed graphically. The relationships among play, games, contests, and spots can be shown in the form of a simple interverted tree diagram.

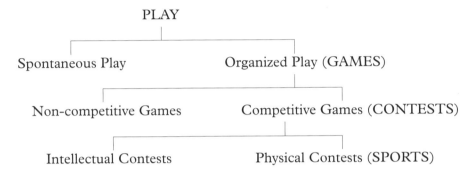

Most scholars, siding with Weber rather than with Wittgenstein, agree that a paradigmatic definition is useful and that it makes sense to consider sports as rule-bound non-utilitarian activities. The most common skirmishes take place around the stipulation that all sports are, by definition, contests. Philosophers, anthropologists, and sociologists have all greatly contributed to the development of sports studies without this emphasis on the distinction between competitive and non-competitive games. For instance, in a subtle book that deserves more attention than it has received, Egon Steinkamp argues that sports are frequently but not invariably characterized by competition.[5] Popular speech bears him out. Noncompetitive recreational cycling, jogging, hiking, and swimming are commonly classified as sports. The counter argument to such expansiveness is pragmatic. Cycling through New England in October, when the leaves have exploded into autumnal color, is physically and mentally totally unlike participating in the Tour de France. Acutely aware of differences of this sort, John Nauright writes that sport is the form of body movement culture that is focused on achievement in a competitive environment. I prefer a simpler formulation: all sports are non-utilitarian physical contests.

One of the advantages of the rather austere ideal-type definition that I have suggested is that it allows for the full range of historical variation. The chariot races at ancient Olympia and the archery contests of Heian Japan, an impromptu race between two six-year-olds and the World Cup – these are vastly different activities with vastly different meanings, but all of them can be seen as nonutilitarian physical contests (at least to the degree that the participants take intrinsic pleasure in the activity). The paradigm is, in other words, the equivalent of a algebraic formula that is capable of describing an infinite number of permutations.

It is important to emphasize that this formulaic definition leaves open the question of meaning. The meanings ascribed to sports vary from time to time, from place to place, and from individual to individual. The marathon race is a good example. The most basic and least debatable "meaning" of a marathon is that someone was able to run 42 kilometers faster than anyone else in the race, but there are a myriad of other possible meanings. Consider the marathon from the spectator's point of view (which is already a significant limitation). When the race was first run, in 1896, it was –among other things –a commemoration of the Athenian military victory over the Persian invaders nearly twenty-four centuries earlier. When the first marathon race was won by Spirdon Louys, a Greek peasant, many spectators, including the Greek royal family, took his victory to mean that modern Greeks were worthy successors of their ancient ancestors. Cultural critics (if there were any among the spectators) may have concluded that peasants, who live close to nature, are more "vital" than "uprooted" urbanites. Nearly a century later, when Joan Benoit won the first-ever women's marathon at the Los Angeles Olympics, feminist spectators seem to have felt that her victory meant – among other things – that the International Olympic Committee had finally acknowledged that female athletes can do anything that male athletes can. Others may have dwelled upon the political implications of yet another American victory at Olympics boycotted by the Soviet Union and most of its allies. In short, the meanings of a sports contest, which are individually as well as socially "constructed", are limited only by the human imagination. And what a sports event means to the participants is presumably as variable as what it means to the spectators. If I am right, then it is foolish to assert, as Brohm does, that sports "imprison" us and equally foolish to assert, as many coaches do, that sports "build character". Specific sports events at specific times and places can do either or neither. Sports events determine winners and losers, but, beyond that, they mean whatever they are made to mean.

If the formulaic abstractness of my paradigm is an advantage, its subjectivity is an obvious drawback. There are clearly practical difficulties with an ideal-type definition that places such great stress upon motivation (intrinsic or extrinsic) and experience (the simple pleasure of physical movement or the complex excitement of a contest). In the real world, motives tend to be mixed (and they probably vary as much as the ascribed meanings do). Students who begin to play volleyball because their physical-education instructor told them it was time to begin to play may or may not have wanted to play. If they did not want to play, then what they do on the volleyball court is work – even if their differently motivated teammates, who were eager to begin, are engaged in play. Linebackers in the National Football League have contractual obligations to do what they do and they are paid large sums of money to do it. They may or may not experience their encounters with the opposition as pleasurable. If they are in the game only for the money, then—for them— it's no game at all. In both cases, and in the case of Nuba wrestlers engaged in a religious ritual, I assume that motivation is mixed and there are likely to be intrinsic as well as extrinsic rewards.

My acknowledgement of the role of subjectivity within my paradigm of sports is very close to Nauright's view. While quite aware of the "commercialisation and professionalisation that [have] beset much of international sport," Nauright argues that there is something about sport that is universal in human experience and imagining. Møller's astute observation about the Neo-Marxists' failure to "make the slightest attempt to understand [the] special attractions that lure athletes to sports" is also apropos. Nauright, Møller, and I seem, therefore, to be at odds with Eichberg. Highly critical of the extreme competitiveness of elite sports, Eichberg has evolved an imaginative taxonomy that enables him, figuratively, to pat the athlete on his or her head and send them off to waste their lives in sports that are part of "the productivism of industrial capitalist society". Displaying the nimbleness of mind that has always characterized his work, Eichberg associates sports with Immanuel Kant's *Kritik der reinen Vernunft* and with Martin Buber's "It", that is, with "a discourse of truth" and with the domain of objective achievement. The contest does determine winners and losers and is in that sense concerned with objective achievement, but sports are obviously about much more than that. Turning away from the subjective experience of sports participants and sports spectators, Eichberg affirms activities that he considers more playful activities. "In pull," writes Eichberg, "I experience *strength* as my strength: 'I can'. Force is felt as physical power, but also as a radiating energy, as my *inner force*." There is no reason to doubt Eichberg's ecstatic experience, but countless athletes have said as much about *their* sports experience. Sports can also be the occasion for the kinds of laughter that Eichberg finds in Inuit games. There are, in fact, carnivalesque sports, such as the "three-legged race", whose main purpose is to provoke hilarity, but these sports are nonetheless sports –as long as the closely bound partners strive to reach the goal before their equally awkward rivals. Like Jean-Marie Brohm, Bero Rigauer, and other Neo-Marxists, Eichberg is unquestionably right to draw attention to the instrumental rationality that is one of the most striking characteristics of modern sports. Instrumental rationality, coupled with the desire to win at all costs, has indeed left little room for the carnivalesque in elite sports, but elite sports are not the whole story. An ideal-type definition of sports, which includes recreational as well as elite sports, children's games as well as the commercialized sports leagues, leaves plenty of room for laughter – and for tears and for every other imaginable form of human response to doing or watching sports.

Aesthetic responses are certainly among the possibilities because the athlete's movements (and the body upon which that movement is inscribed) are frequently perceived to be beautiful. No one who has paid even minimal attention to sports has failed to notice that the figure skaters who compete at the Olympic Games perform dance-like movements accompanied by music. When the element of competition is removed, as it is in the Icecapades and other show-biz exhibitions, the performance *is* a dance – *tout court*. To say this, however, is not quite to say, as Møller does, that sports "can be understood as essentially an aesthetic phenomenon" and that there is "an invisible bond between beauty and efficiency."[6] Sports *can* be an aesthetic phenomenon and efficient movements *can* be beautiful, but no one ever called Emil Zatopek a graceful runner and sumo wrestlers are customarily thought to be ungainly if not positively grotesque. Anna Kornikova is not and probably never will the top player in women's tennis because she routinely loses to less conventionally beautiful players who have a better tennis game. In short, I agree with David Best that beauty is incidental. Møller is correct to argue that the "sport-art analogy can be taken [farther] than the sport-work analogy" because art can also be considered, in an ideal-type definition, as a nonutilitarian activity (*l'art pour l'art*), but the analogy is only an analogy. In the last analysis, sports are *sui generis* and not a subcategory of art. To remove the element of competition from the most breathtakingly beautiful performance of men's diving or women's gymnastics is to remove the activity from the domain of sports.

For me, the most interesting development in the history of sports is the emergence of modern sports in eighteenth-century England and their subsequent diffusion from Europe and North America to the rest of the world. In the effort to delineate the differences between pre-modern and modern sports, Eichberg and I came to some rather similar conclusions, which is partially explained by the fact that I was enormously impressed by his early work. My formulation of the differences focused on seven systematically related formal-structural characteristics: secularism, equality, rationalization, specialization, bureaucratization, quantification, and the quest for records. If I were to reformulate my views today, I'd probably consider specialization and bureaucratization as subcategories of rationalization, but a modification of this sort does not change the argument about the nature of the differences between the past and the present. Nielsen's commentary on the role of gymnastics and modern sports in the development of Finnish national identity refers to a textbook case of the tension between two very different kinds of "body culture".

In my terms, Bale's assertion that the "essence of sport is that it is 'placeless'" is too specific, too focused on one aspect of modern sports. "Placelessness" is a common but certainly not an essential characteristic of modern sports. Bale asserts, "The 'production' of a record *requires* placelessness", but this is overstatement. Standardized space is clearly not a pre-requisite for the establishment of a sports record – as demonstrated by the plethora of records set in dozens of differently configured baseball stadia. To the possible objection that baseball records are not "true" records because the stadia differ, one can reply that track-and-field records are also suspect because 400-meter tracks also differ. Absolute placelessness is unattainable. While Bale's analysis of "placelessness" is not an adequate statement of the essence of sport (and was probably not meant as an adequate statement), it does provide new insights into the powerful tendency of modern sports to standardize (i.e., rationalize) space in an effort to equalize the conditions of competition. Seen in this light, the quest for "placelessness" is the spatial equivalent of the weight classes that provide a modicum of equality in *Schwerathletik* (e.g., boxing, wrestling, judo, weight-lifting). The equivalent label, "weightlessness", does not, however, seem appropriate for sports whose heaviest proponents are dauntingly massive.

Hoberman's discussion of performance-enhancing drugs in the world of professional cycling is not explicitly a commentary on the essence of sports, but his analysis sheds additional light on the nature of modern sports. That intense competition tempts athletes to cheat, to violate the rules, is not exactly news. The ancient Olympics had officials whose role was to detect and punish the cheaters. What Hoberman shows, expanding upon some insights from Møller's earlier work, is that cyclists who decide to "dope" themselves do so in order to restore equality destroyed by those who had been taking performance-enhancing drugs. Ironically, fairness dictates that every cyclist take drugs if one cyclist does.

Hoberman's essay is also valuable for its insights into the attractiveness of risk. The possibility of death, which certainly pervaded the Roman arena when gladiator met gladiator, hovers in the background of the Tour de France. The motives behind sports participation, like the significance ascribed to it, are many and varied. None – not even the euphoria associated with the perfect move or the perfect play – can be isolated as the "essence of sport". We are left – in my opinion – with an ideal-type definition, with "nonutilitarian physical contests". We are left with an infinite number of sports and sports contests, each of which has to be understood as socially and individually constructed. Small wonder that historians disagree in their interpretations of the toxophilic talents of Amenophis III and the political significance of the 1998 Tour de France. Like algebra, my ideal-type definition is formulaic and abstract, but that is its advantage. Of what use is an algebraic formula in which "x" is always equal to 8.5?

Notes

1. Ludwig Wittgenstein, *Schriften: Philosophe Untersuchungen* (Frankfurt a.M.: Suhrkamp, 1960), p. 324. The discussion of the concept of "*Spiel*" covers pp. 325-26.
2. Max Weber, *Wirtschaft und Gesellschaft*, ed. Johannes Winckelmann, 2 vols. (Cologne: Kiepenheuer & Witsch, 1964): 1:15.
3. Marjatta Marin, "Gender-Differences in Sport and Movement in Finland", *International Review of Sport Sociology*, 23:4 (1988): 345-58.
4. An example of the last occurs when I try to run faster today than I did yesterday.
5. Egon Steinkamp, *Was ist eigentlich Sport?* (Wuppertal: Hans Putty, 1983).
6. Møller might have cited another author who tries valiently to classify sports among the fine arts; see Pierre Frayssinet, *Le Sport parmi les beaux-arts* (Paris: Dargaud, 1968).

The authors

John Bale is professor, Ph.D. and teaches and researches at Aarhus University, Denmark and Keele University, UK. He has pioneered the geographical study of sport and is the author of many articles and several books, of which *Imagined Olympians – Body Culture and Colonial Representation in Rwanda* (2002) is the latest.

Henning Eichberg, Dr. phil. Habil, is cultural sociologist and historian, working as research fellow at the Research Institute for Sport, Culture and Civil Society (IFO) in Gerlev, Denmark. Formerly professor at the Universities of Odense and Copenhagen, he has also lectured at universities in Austria (Graz, Salzburg, Vienna), Finland (Jyväskylä), England (Keele), France (Rennes 2), Germany (Free University Berlin, Tübingen, Vechta/Osnabrück), Japan (Tsukuba, Kyoto) and Sweden (Lund). In 1987, he co-founded the Institut International d'Anthropologie Corporelle (Rennes/France).

He has published more than 30 books in various fields: the history and cultural sociology of body culture and sport; the cultural ecology of movement; the history of early modern military technology; Indonesian studies; studies in democracy, ethnic minorities and national identity. Among these are *Der Weg des Sports in die industrielle Zivilisation* (1973), *Militär und Technik* (1976), *Leistung, Spannung, Geschwindigkeit* (1978), *Festung, Zentralmacht und Sozialgeometrie* (1989) and *Body Cultures* (1998).

Allen Guttmann is the author of *From Ritual to Record* (1978) and eight other books of sports history, the most recent of which, coauthored with Lee Thompson, is *Japanese Sports* (2001). With Karen Christensen and Gertrud Pfister, he has edited the 3-volume *International Encyclopedia of Women and Sport* (2000). His books have received awards from the US Olympic Committee, the North American Society for Sports History, the International Society for the History of Physical Education and Sport, and the International Olympic Committee. He teaches at Amherst College Massachusetts USA and has been a visiting professor at a number of American, European, and Japanese universities, including the Deutsche Sporthochschule.

John Hoberman has been active in sports studies for the past 25 years as a scholar and journalist. He is the author of *Sport and Political Ideology* (1984), *The Olympic Crisis: Sport, Politics and the Moral Order* (1986), *Mortal Engines: The Science of Performance and the Dehumanization of Sport* (1992), *Darwin's Athletes: How Sport Has Damaged Black America and Preserved the Myth of Race* (1997), and *Testosterone Dreams: Rejuvenation, Aphrodisia, Doping* (forthcoming). He is Professor of Germanic Studies at the University of Texas at Austin, Texas, and Visiting Professor at the University of Southern Denmark (Odense).

Verner Møller is associate professor at the Institute of Sport Science & Clinical Biomechanics, in the Faculty of Health Sciences at the University of Southern Denmark. He has edited and written books on sports, health and doping one of which, *Dopingdjævlen* ("The Doping Devil"), is in the process of being translated into English. His main field of research is body culture, health, drugs, and elite sports.

John Nauright is professor of Sport and Leisure Studies and Director of the Abertay Sport and Leisure Research Group and Golf Research Unit at the University of Abertay Dundee in Scotland. He is also co-coordinator of the Northeast Scotland Tourism Research Network, a director of the Dundee Ice Arena and member of the Institute of Commonwealth Studies at the University of London. He has been Visiting Professor at the Universities of Southern Denmark (Odense) and Copenhagen and has been invited as a visiting professor to the Lakshimibai National Institute of Physical Education in India. He is the author or editor of nine books in sports studies including *Sport, Cultures and Identities in South Africa*; *Making Men: Rugby and Masculine Identity* (with Timothy Chandler); and *The Political Economy of Sport* (with Kimberly Schimmel). He is editor of the academic journals *Football Studies* and *International Sports Studies* and consulting editor of the *Journal of Physical Education and Sports Sciences*. His current research focuses on race and sport in the USA and South Africa; the international expansion of golf in the early twentieth century; and bids for major events.

Niels Kayser Nielsen is senior lecturer at Department of History, Aarhus University. He has published several books and articles on nationalism, sports history, body culture, food sociology, british social and cultural history. His current research focuses on food and taste, Nordic history in the 19th and 20th century and Eastern Europe's history 1914-1948.